ASSESSING MENTAL HEALTH AND PSYCHOSOCIAL NEEDS AND RESOURCES

Toolkit for humanitarian settings

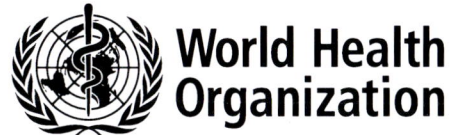

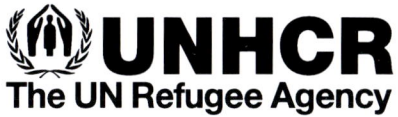

Preface

While mental health and psychosocial problems are common in all communities of the world, these problems are much more frequent among people who have faced adversity, such as exposure to a humanitarian crisis. A key element of responding to these problems is a better understanding of needs and resources. WHO and UNHCR receive frequent requests from the field to advise on assessment of mental health and psychosocial issues in humanitarian settings.

Mental health and psychosocial support (MHPSS) is a term used to describe a wide range of actions that address social, psychological and psychiatric problems that are either pre-existing or emergency-induced. These actions are carried out in highly different contexts by organizations and people with different professional backgrounds, in different sectors and with different types of resources. All these different actors – and their donors – need practical assessments leading to recommendations that can be used immediately to improve people's mental health and well-being.

Although a range of assessment tools exist, what has been missing is an overall approach that clarifies when to use which tool for what purpose. This document offers an approach to assessment that should help you review information that is already available and only collect new data that will be of practical use, depending on your capacity and the phase of the humanitarian crisis.

This document is rooted in two policy documents, the IASC Reference Group's (2010) *Mental Health and Psychosocial Support in Humanitarian Emergencies: What Should Humanitarian Health Actors Know?* and the Sphere Handbook's Standard on Mental Health (Sphere Project, 2011).

This document is written primarily for public health actors. As the social determinants of mental health and psychosocial problems occur across sectors, half of the tools in the accompanying toolkit cover MHPSS assessment issues relevant to other sectors as well as the health sector.

This document should help you to collect the necessary information to assist people affected by humanitarian crises more effectively.

Shekhar Saxena

Director
Department of Mental Health
and Substance Abuse
WHO, Geneva

Steve Corliss

Director
Division of Programme
Support and Management
UNHCR, Geneva

Acknowledgements

This joint project between WHO and UNHCR was coordinated by Mark van Ommeren (Department of Mental Health and Substance Abuse, WHO). The work was supervised by Shekhar Saxena (Director, Department of Mental Health and Substance Abuse, WHO) and Marian Schilperoord (Chief, Public Health and HIV Section, UNHCR).

The document was written by Wietse A. Tol (Johns Hopkins University School of Public Health) and Mark van Ommeren (WHO).

We are pleased to acknowledge UNHCR for early testing of selected tools in this document.

We are grateful to the following people for peer review or testing of one or more of the new tools in this document: Jonathan Abrahams (WHO), Alastair Ager (Colombia University), Heni Anastasia (Christian World Services), Giuseppe Annunziata (WHO), Nancy Baron (Global Psycho-Social Initiative), Anja Baumann (WHO), Theresa Betancourt (Harvard University), Cecile Bizouerne (Action Contre le Faim), Paul Bolton (Johns Hopkins University), Maria Bray (Terre des Hommes), Jorge Castilla (European Community Humanitarian Office), Joseph Coyne (University of Pennsylvania), Nathalie Drew (WHO), Carolina Echeverri (UNHCR consultant), Tonka Elbs (CARE Austria), Rabih El Chammay (consultant), Richard Garfield (Colombia University), Rita Giacaman (Birzeit University), Jane Gilbert (consultant), Andre Griekspoor (WHO), Sarah Harrison (Church of Sweden), Lynne Jones (consultant), Mark Jordans (HealthNet TPO), Devora Kestel (WHO/PAHO), Albert Maramis (WHO), Anita Marini (WHO), Amanda Melville (UNICEF), Ken Miller (consultant), Matthijs Muijen (WHO), Bhava Nath Poudyal (consultant), Ruth O'Connell (UNICEF), Pau Perez-Sales (MdM-Spain), Sabine Rakatomalala (Terre des Hommes), Khalid Saeed (WHO), Benedetto Saraceno (Nova University of Lisbon), Norman Sartorius (Association for the Improvement of Mental Health Programmes), Alison Schafer (World Vision International), Maya Semrau (Institute of Psychiatry King's College London), Derrick Silove (University of New South Wales), Mike Slade (Institute of Psychiatry King's College London), Leslie Snider (War Trauma Foundation), Egbert Sondorp (London School of Hygiene and Tropical Medicine), Renato Souza (International Committee of the Red Cross), Lindsay Stark (Colombia University), Emmanuel Streel (UNICEF), Marian Tankink (HealthNet TPO), Matthias Themel (European Commission), Graham Thornicroft (Institute of Psychiatry King's College London), Liv Torheim (FAFO), Peter Ventevogel (HealthNet TPO), Kristian Wahlbeck (WHO), Inka Weissbecker (International Medical Corps), Michael Wessells (Colombia University), and Nana Wiedemann (International Federation of Red Cross and Red Crescent Societies).

Table of Contents

Preface — 3

Acknowledgements — 4

A quick guide to identifying tools — 7

1. Introduction — 8
- 1.1 How to use this toolkit? — 8
- 1.2 Who should use the toolkit? — 9
- 1.3 How was the toolkit developed? — 10
- 1.4 Culture and mental health — 10

2. Overview of the assessment process — 11

3. Assessment methodology — 14
- 3.1 Selecting assessment topics and tools from this toolkit — 14
- 3.2 Estimating the prevalence of mental health problems — 17
- 3.3 Collecting qualitative and quantitative data — 19

4. Translating assessment into action — 25
- 4.1 Drafting a report with recommendations — 25
- 4.2 Communicating recommendations — 26

Tools 1 to 12 (see quick guide on page 7 or back page for page numbers) — 29

Bibliography — 78

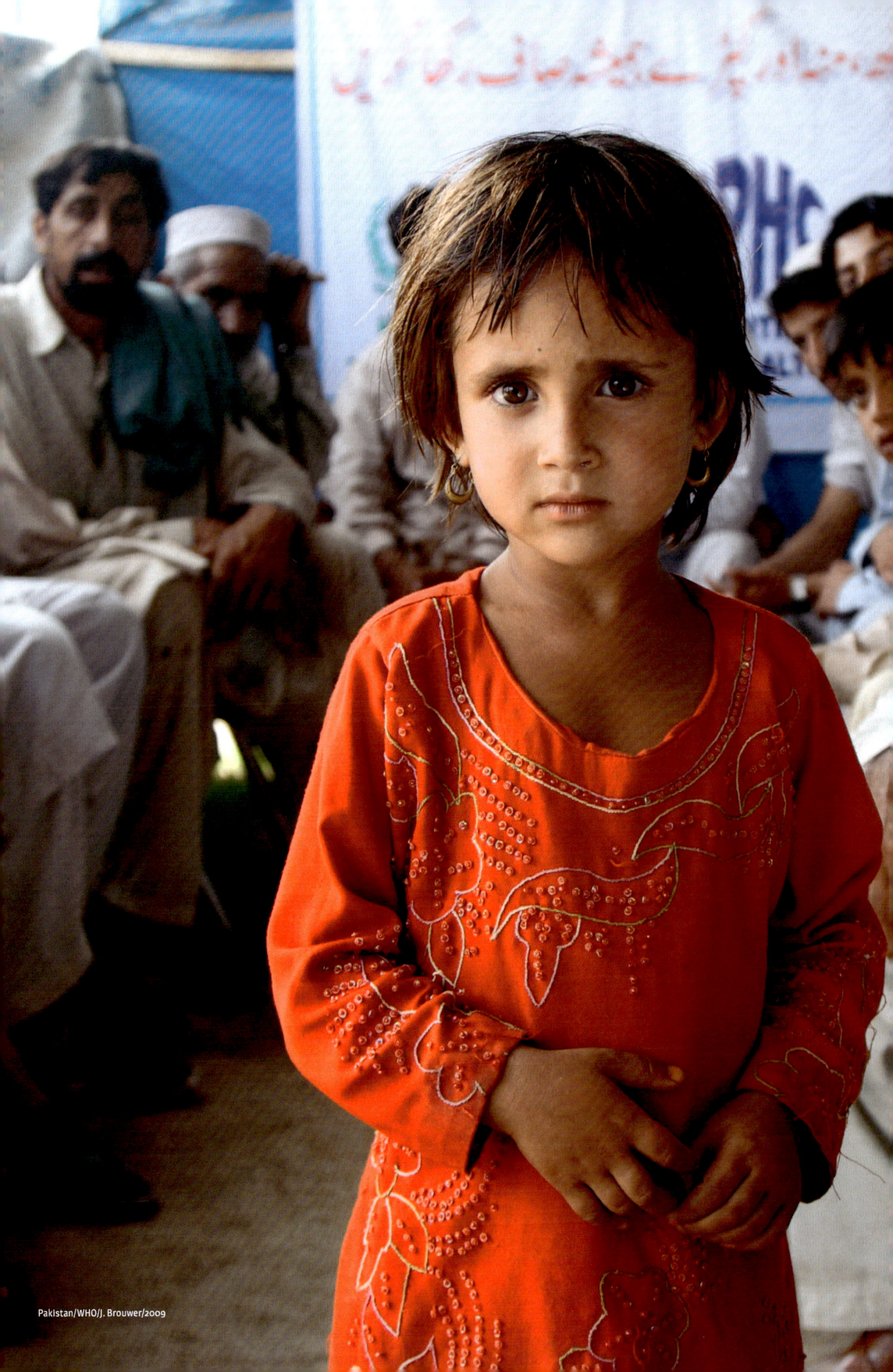

Pakistan/WHO/J. Brouwer/2009

A quick guide to identifying tools

Tool #	Title	Method	Why use this tool	Page
For coordination and advocacy				
1	Who is Where, When, doing What (4Ws) in Mental Health and Psychosocial Support (MHPSS): summary of manual with activity codes	Interviews with agency programme managers	For coordination, through mapping what mental health and psychosocial supports are available	30
2	WHO-UNHCR Assessment Schedule of Serious Symptoms in Humanitarian Settings (WASSS)	Part of a community household survey (representative sample)	For advocacy, by showing the prevalence of mental health problems in the community	34
3	Humanitarian Emergency Setting Perceived Needs Scale (HESPER)	Part of a community household survey (representative sample) Or, exceptionally (in acute, major emergencies) as a convenience sample	For informing response, through collecting data on the frequency of physical, social, and psychological perceived needs in the community	41
For MHPSS through health services				
4	Checklist for site visits at institutions in humanitarian settings	Site visits and interviews with staff and patients	For protection and care for people with mental or neurological disabilities in institutions	42
5	Checklist for integrating mental health in primary health care (PHC) in humanitarian settings	Site visits and interviews with primary health care programme managers	For planning a mental health response in PHC	47
6	Neuropsychiatric component of the Health Information System (HIS)	Clinical epidemiology using the HIS	For advocacy and for planning and monitoring a mental health response in PHC	53
7	Template to assess mental health system formal resources in humanitarian settings	Review of documents and interviews with managers of services	For planning of (early) recovery and reconstruction, through knowing the formal resources in the regional/national mental health system	55
For MHPSS through different sectors, including through community support				
8	Checklist on obtaining general (non-MHPSS specific) information from sector leads	Review of available documents	For summarizing general (non-MHPSS specific) information already known about the current humanitarian emergency (to avoid collecting data on issues that are already known)	59
9	Template for desk review of pre-existing information relevant to MHPSS in the region/country	Literature review	For summarizing MHPSS information about this region/country - already known before the current humanitarian emergency (to avoid collecting data on issues that are already known)	60
10	Participatory assessment: perceptions by general community members	Interviews with general community members (free listing with further questions)	For learning about local perspectives on problems and coping to develop an appropriate MHPSS response	63
11	Participatory assessment: perceptions by community members with in-depth knowledge of the community	Interviews with key informants or groups		70
12	Participatory assessment: perceptions by severely affected people	Interviews with severely affected people (free listing with further questions)		74

Note: MHPSS indicates mental health and psychosocial support.

1. Introduction

1.1 HOW TO USE THIS TOOLKIT?

This document provides an approach and a toolkit to help those designing and conducting an assessment of mental health and psychosocial needs and resources in major humanitarian crises. These could include major natural and human-made disasters and complex emergencies (for example armed conflicts).

In general, assessments are aimed at:
- providing a broad understanding of the humanitarian situation;
- analysing people's problems and their ability to deal with them; and
- analysing resources to decide, in consultation with stakeholders, the nature of any response required.

Assessments are also helpful to start engagement with stakeholders, including governments, community stakeholders and national and international agencies.

The IASC (2007) Guidelines on Mental Health and Psychosocial Support in Emergency Settings suggest topics that should be covered in assessments of mental health and psychosocial issues. However, these guidelines do not offer guidance on **how** to collect the data or what information is typically needed for what health-sector actions. This document – written mainly for humanitarian actors in the health sector - is intended to help fill these gaps.

This document is rooted in two policy documents, the IASC Reference Group's (2010) *Mental Health and Psychosocial Support in Humanitarian Emergencies: What Should Humanitarian Health Actors Know?* and the Sphere Handbook's Standard on Mental Health (Sphere Project, 2011).

Page 7 (and the back cover) of this document provides a quick guide to identify tools and shows how the tools in this toolkit are linked to the main recommended health-sector actions in the area of mental health and psychosocial support (MHPSS).

Because of the broad scope of assessment topics, assessments should, as far as possible, be a coordinated effort. They greatly benefit from collaboration between partners. For guidance on coordinated assessments, see the work by the IASC Task Force on Needs Assessment (IASC NATF, 2011).

There is no 'one assessment that fits all'. This document is not a cookbook. Rather, it provides a toolkit and an approach to selecting the right tools. You should select a few tools and adapt them within each assessment project and specific situation, depending on what you want the assessment to achieve.

Assessment objectives depend on:
- what information is already available;
- the phase of the emergency; and
- the abilities, resources and interests of the assessment team.

The approach in this document – in line with recent interagency recommendations (IASC NATF 2011, IASC 2012) - covers collecting both primary data (new data) as well as secondary data (existing data).

1.2 WHO SHOULD USE THE TOOLKIT?

While this document is written primarily for public health agencies, many of the assessment tools presented are very relevant for staff working in other sectors. Health actors may work at any of the following different levels of the health system:
- in the community (for example at people's homes);
- in first-level and second-level health facilities (for example primary health care clinics, policlinics, general hospitals); and
- in tertiary care (for example mental hospitals).

As the social conditions that contribute to mental health and psychosocial problems occur across all sectors, approximately half of the tools in this document cover MHPSS assessment issues that are relevant to other sectors as well as the health sector.

This document assumes you know about mental health and psychosocial concepts as outlined in the IASC MHPSS Guidelines (2007). Although some explanations are given in the text, this document also assumes you have a basic knowledge of assessment techniques, for example, how to:
- conduct, analyse and report on semi-structured key informant interviews and group interviews;
- conduct, analyse and report on surveys; and
- manage the logistics of an assessment, budget, and train data collectors and so on.

Much of the rigour and quality of the assessment will depend on the abilities of the assessment team leader and their team. At a minimum, assessment team leaders should have previous experience in designing, conducting, analysing, and reporting on qualitative and quantitative assessment methods in humanitarian settings. Team members should bring together good knowledge of:

- the socio-cultural context in which the humanitarian crisis takes place; and
- mental health issues and programming in humanitarian settings.

1.3. HOW WAS THE TOOLKIT DEVELOPED?

The toolkit was developed through an iterative process that involved consulting experts, holding multiple rounds of peer review, and pilot testing of various tools. Development started with a list of all the different assessment topics recommended in the IASC MHPSS Guidelines' Action Sheet on assessment. Possible questions (with defined assessment techniques and target respondents) on each of these topics were then entered into a large table. As much as possible, previously tested questions and tools were entered into the table. Subsequently, questions were grouped together across topics, according to assessment technique and type of respondent. Duplicate and superfluous questions were removed. Questions that had no obvious relationship to health-sector action were also removed. The grouped questions were then converted into assessment tools, each with an explicit objective that relates to one of the key actions listed in the revised Mental Health Standard of the 2011 Sphere Handbook. The IASC Reference Group on MHPSS reviewed a few tools involving assessment which crossed a number of sectors (Tools 1, 9, 10, 11) and this resulted in the Reference Group adopting these four tools.

1.4. CULTURE AND MENTAL HEALTH

Assessment coordinators will always be challenged to find a balance between obtaining:
- quick and practical information (through, for example, rapid assessments of main issues to start service delivery); and
- knowledge of the very complex socio-cultural reality (through, for example, in-depth ethnographic assessments).

Unfortunately, there is no easy answer to achieving this balance.

Cultural dimensions of care in this toolkit are addressed in a number of ways, including:
- a template for literature reviews of the relevant social science and medical literature which apply to the specific context; and
- assessment tools that rapidly collect perspectives of local community members and other stakeholders with regard to mental health and psychosocial support.

It will be important to keep in mind that the tools in this toolkit generally provide rapid and superficial answers to complex questions. Information collected with these tools will require critical reflection and, where the situation evolves, further data collection.

2. Overview of the assessment process

Assessing needs is a continuous process. Figure 2.1 below depicts this continuous process and outlines the different steps involved in assessing needs.

Before starting any assessments it is crucial to coordinate with the relevant stakeholders, including, as appropriate, the government, sector leads, representatives of the target group, and other humanitarian actors.

It is advisable to coordinate assessments (for example dividing topics or geographical areas between humanitarian agencies) for a number of reasons, including:
- to make efficient use of resources;
- to gain a more complete picture of needs;
- to avoid asking the same questions to the same participants.

If you are an agency from outside, you should try to coordinate assessments with local researchers and make use of existing government and university capabilities.

It is highly recommended that agencies planning to carry out coordinated MHPSS assessments apply the operational guidance on coordinated needs assessment by the IASC NATF, 2011.

The approach of this toolkit on mental health and psychosocial support needs and resources involves the following four types of data collection:
- Literature review (Tool 9).
- Collecting existing information from relevant stakeholders, including government (for example, Tools 7 and 8).
- Gathering new information through adding questions about psychosocial and mental health concerns to general health, nutrition, protection or other assessments done by non-MHPSS actors[1] (for example, Tool 2 may be added to such assessments).
- Filling in any gaps in knowledge by collecting new information on mental health and psychosocial issues through specific MHPSS assessment including, for example, interviews and site visits, surveys, and group and key informant interviews (for example, Tool 11).

---

1   Ideally, integrating relevant questions in assessment formats is done while preparing for emergencies, that is before they occur.

FIGURE 2.1   FLOW CHART OF NEEDS ASSESSMENT

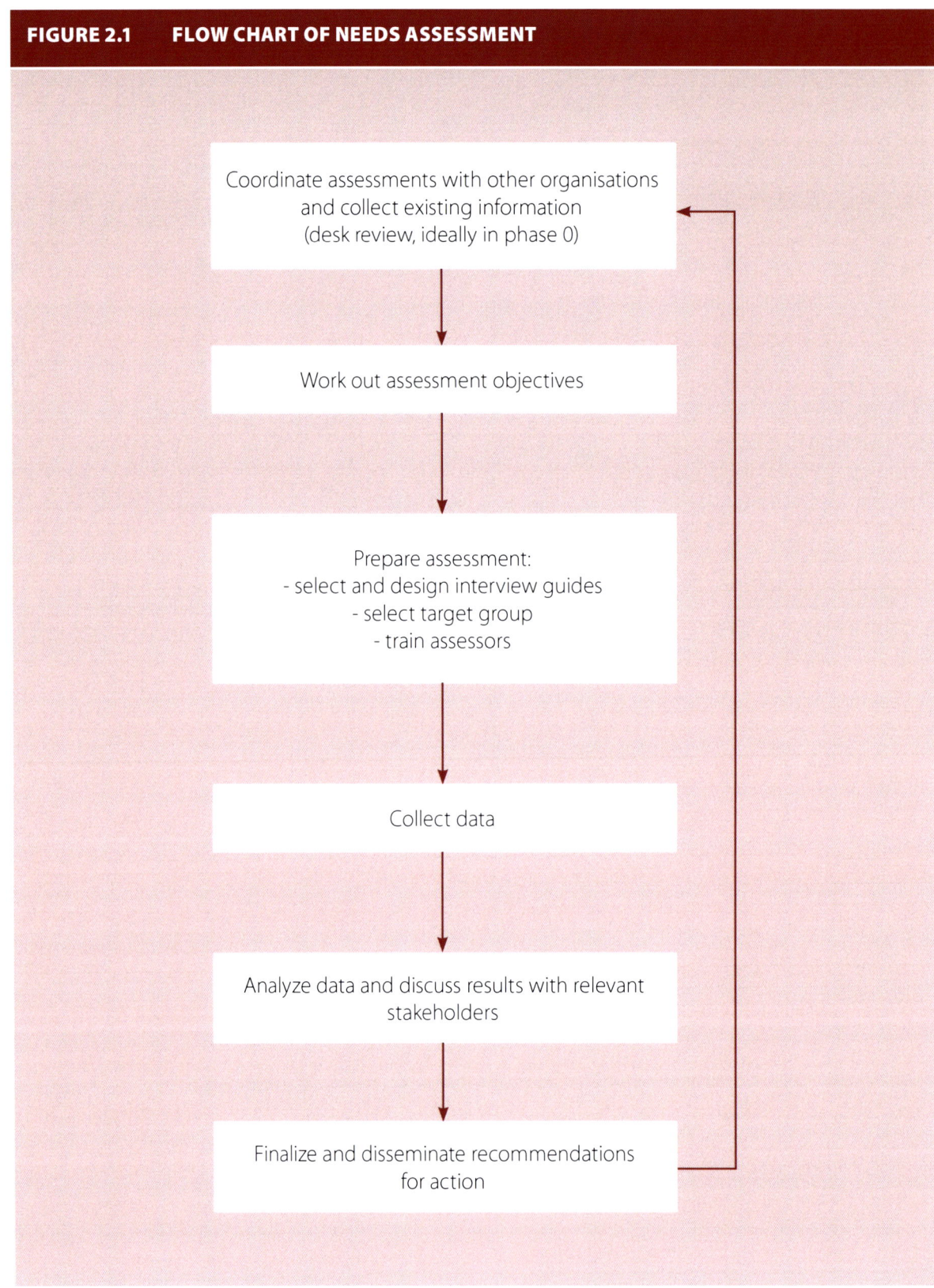

TABLE 2.1	GOOD PRACTICE PRINCIPLES FOR ASSESSMENT

1. Make sure to **coordinate with relevant stakeholders** (including, where possible, governments, NGOs, community and religious organisations, local universities and affected populations) and have them participate in designing the assessment; interpreting the results; and translating results into recommendations.

2. **Include different sections** of the affected population, paying attention to children, youth, women, men, elderly people and different cultural, religious and socio-economic groups.

3. **Design** and analyse assessments with a focus on action, rather than on collecting information only. Collecting too much data (that is, so much data that you cannot analyse it all or meaningfully use it) wastes resources and places unnecessary burdens on interviewees.

4. **Attention to conflict**, for example by maintaining impartiality and independence, considering possible tensions and not putting people at risk by asking questions.

5. Be aware that the assessment methodology and behaviour of the assessment team members are appropriate to the local **culture**.

6. **Assess both needs *and* resources** to increase the likelihood that any humanitarian response builds on the supports and resources that are already there.

7. Be aware of **ethical principles**, including respecting privacy, confidentiality, informed and voluntary participation, and the best interest of the interviewee (see section 3.3 on informed consent below).

8. **Assessment teams** should be trained in ethical principles and basic interviewing skills. They should be knowledgeable about the local context and balanced in terms of gender. Some of the team members should be themselves members of (or very familiar with) the local population. They should know about referral sources.

9. **Data collection methods** can include literature review, group interviews, key informant interviews, observation and site visits.

10. Assessments should be **timely** so they are tailored to the phase of the humanitarian crisis, with more detailed assessments taking place in later phases.

3. Assessment methodology

3.1 SELECTING ASSESSMENT TOPICS AND TOOLS FROM THIS TOOLKIT

Assessments usually need to focus on a selected number of topics and tools. The quick guide on page 7 and the back cover of this document gives a list of potential key actions for health agencies in the area of mental health and psychosocial support. This list covers all but one of the key actions in the Sphere Handbook Mental Health Standard (Sphere Project, 2011).[2] For each key action mentioned there are one or more assessment tools in this toolkit.

When selecting tools from this toolkit, it is important to keep the following in mind:

1. **Develop a clear framework and objectives of your assessment**. This will help you to prioritise the information you need and guide your selection of the tools.

2. **Remember that time is short and resources are limited.** Do not burden affected people unnecessarily; a study of already available information is crucial to minimise the topics for further assessment. There is no point in collecting the same information twice unless there is doubt whether existing information is up-to-date or of sufficient quality. Only collect information that can lead to humanitarian action.

3. **There is rarely a need for in-depth information on all topics**. The information needed depends on an agency's mandate and ability to act on the assessment. When assessments become too broad, it is difficult to collect, analyse and report good quality information.

4. **Collaboration is helpful.** When inter-agency (coordinated) assessments are done, the burden of doing assessments can be shared across agencies. Such assessments are recommended because they tend to be more credible, and they tend to support collaborative planning (IASC NATF, 2011). Agencies can divide topics and select a number of more specific topics according to their strengths.

5. **Collecting information from different types of sources provides a bigger picture** (cf. IASC NATF, 2011). This toolkit contains tools for the following sources.
   - Perceptions by interviewees of themselves (Tool 2, part A; Tool 12)
   - Perceptions by interviewees of others (Tool 2, part B; Tools 10, 11)
   - Perceptions by interviewees of themselves and others (Tool 3)
   - Health information system data (Tool 6)
   - Services offered by agencies (Tools 1, 4, 5, 7)
   - Secondary data on an affected area as a whole (Tools 8, 9)

6. **Plan to evaluate the validity of collected information.** Choices for methodology should be based on:
   - available resources (skills, time, money); and
   - the decision to check the validity of findings by collecting related information in more than one way (triangulation).

---

[2] The only Sphere key action that is not reflected in this toolkit is the one on addressing alcohol and drug use, because assessment of alcohol and substance use issues has been covered previously in a UNHCR/WHO publication (2008). The previous publication thus complements this toolkit.

For example, you can compare data from the desk literature review with information obtained during a site visit and responses from communities about the need for care.

This document sometimes provides more than one method to assess an issue, and you should select the methods most appropriate and feasible for you. Checking primary data (new data) with secondary data (existing data) is an efficient form of triangulation.

Figure 3.1 shows the process of choosing assessment topics and methodology. After selecting topics and methodology, you can estimate the time and human resources needed for your assessment. You can adapt the selected tools to the context and the purpose of the assessment. For a good example of how you can adapt and use the tools in this kit, see the IMC (2011) assessment in Libya.

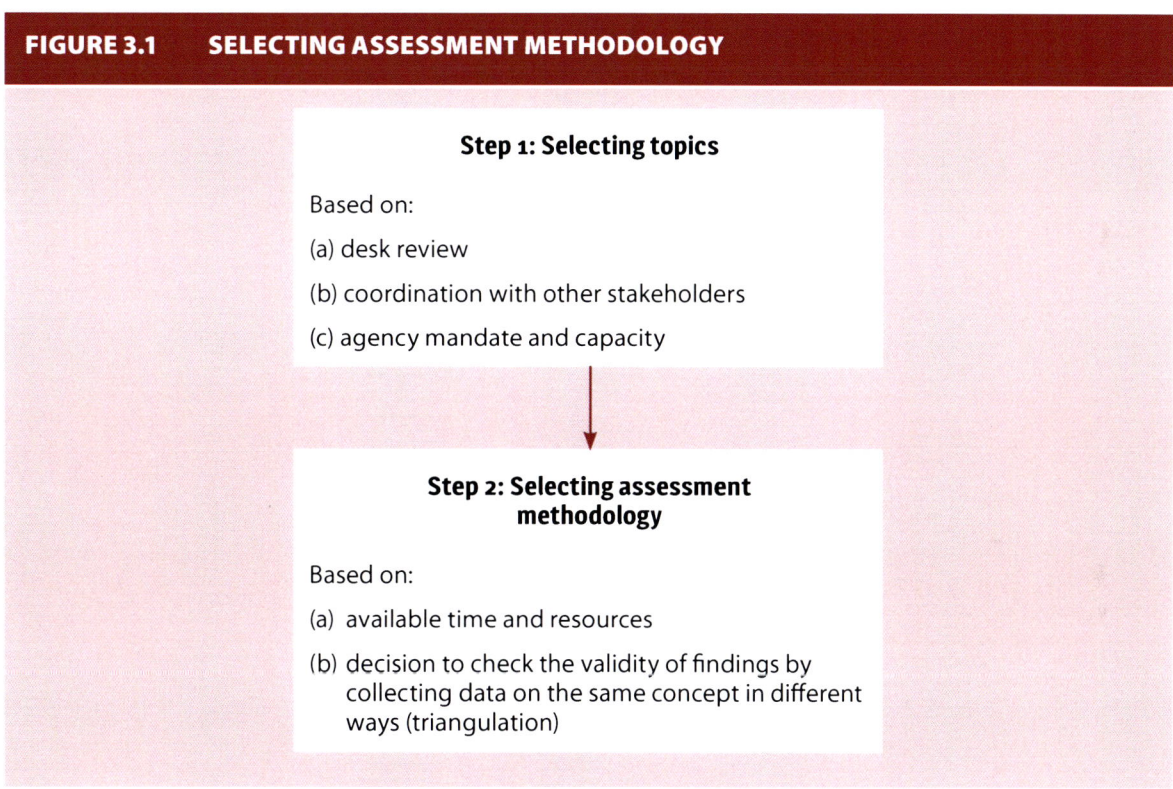

FIGURE 3.1 SELECTING ASSESSMENT METHODOLOGY

Step 1: Selecting topics

Based on:

(a) desk review

(b) coordination with other stakeholders

(c) agency mandate and capacity

Step 2: Selecting assessment methodology

Based on:

(a) available time and resources

(b) decision to check the validity of findings by collecting data on the same concept in different ways (triangulation)

There is no strict 1:1 relationship between the phase of a crisis and the use of specific assessment tools. However, the following guidance may be given.

Within the international humanitarian response system, agencies increasingly discuss assessment in terms of four phases explained in Table 3.1.

TABLE 3.1	PHASES, TIME FRAMES AND THE AMOUNT OF ATTENTION PAID TO MENTAL HEALTH IN ASSESSMENTS OF MAJOR SUDDEN-ONSET CRISES
Phases with examples of time frame after start of major sudden-onset crisis (as suggested by the IASC NATF (2011))[3]	**Use of tools in this toolkit**
Phase 0 (before the sudden-onset crisis)	Conduct a desk review (Tool 9) and identify available services and actors (Tool 1). If resources are available, conduct an in-depth assessment focused on mental health and psychosocial wellbeing as it applies to the health sector (use any of the tools in this kit).
Phase 1 (for example, the first 72 hours of a sudden-onset crisis)	Initiate or update a desk review (Tool 9). Review projections on mental disorders based on knowledge of previous crises (for example, see Table 3.2). Set up an assessment of basic survival, protection and care of people in institutions (Tool 4).
Phase 2 (for example, the first two weeks of a sudden-onset crisis)	Include a few questions on mental health problems (for example, on care for people in institutions) as part of any Multi cluster/sector Initial Rapid Assessment (MIRA; IASC, 2012) and consider using the Humanitarian Emergency Setting Perceived Needs Scale (HESPER, Tool 3) in a convenience sample. Set up participatory assessments to develop mental health and psychosocial support (for example, Tools 10 to 12).
Phase 3 (for example, weeks 3 and 4 after a sudden-onset crisis)	Include a subsection on mental and social aspects of health within general health assessments (for example, Tools 2, 4, 5, 6). Prepare in-depth assessment on mental health and psychosocial wellbeing (any of the tools in this kit).
Phase 4 (the remaining time)	Assess resources in the formal mental health system (Tool 7) to inform recovery activities. Conduct an in-depth assessment focused on mental health and psychosocial wellbeing (any of the tools in this kit).

With regard to these four phases, you should note the following:
- Although imperfect, this common language on the order of phases and tasks is useful for communicating and collaborative planning.
- The time frames in Table 3.1 above vary with the scale and severity of humanitarian crises and with the ability to respond.
- You need to complete, analyse and report rapidly on all assessments in phases 1 to 3 for them to be meaningful, because the situation on the ground can change quickly.

---

[3] There is no full agreement on the time-lines suggested, which apply only to sudden-onset emergencies. Each of the phases will take longer when the onset is slow. Also, phase 3 may take much longer (for example, up to the end of the 3rd month if the emergency is particularly severe or when access is poor).

- In general the greater part of humanitarian assistance (including almost all support in complex emergencies) is provided in phase 4.
- Most mental health assessments tend to take place in phase 4.
- Where possible, you should avoid vertical (stand-alone) mental health assessments in phases 1 to 3. You should include them in multi- sector or health-sector assessments.
- If an area has only recently opened after a longer time period (for example, because of security) you should start assessment in phase 1.

Most of the tools and questions covered in this document are for phase 4. Yet you can apply tools in earlier phases as part of multi-sector and health-sector assessments as follows:
- You can usually ask questions on perceived needs through the Humanitarian Emergency Setting Perceived Needs Scale (HESPER[4], Tool 3) in convenience samples as early as phase 2. At the time of writing, the HESPER questions are the base of the draft primary data collection questions in phase 2 of the IASC's Multi cluster/sector Initial Rapid Assessment (MIRA; IASC, 2012).[5]
- Tool 4 (on institutions) applies from the beginning of the emergency, because a key question is whether people in mental hospitals or other institutions (for example, old age homes, orphanages and prisons) have been forgotten or abandoned without access to clean water, food, physical health care or protection from violence and abuse. Given that people in mental hospitals are too often forgotten, advocacy is needed to make sure that any MIRA assessment automatically also occurs in institutions.
- You can add questions on serious symptoms of distress (see Tool 2) to population-based general health surveys (phase 3).
- You should add mental health categories (see Tool 6) to the health information system (HIS) (phase 3).

3.2 ESTIMATING THE PREVALENCE OF MENTAL HEALTH PROBLEMS

Attempts to estimate the prevalence of various mental disorders have been common. This document, however, does not cover surveys on the prevalence of mental disorders (that is, psychiatric epidemiology). Such surveys can be important for advocacy and academic value but, more often than not, are of limited practical value when designing a humanitarian response. Also, such surveys are very challenging to conduct in a meaningful manner in humanitarian settings. Surveys of mental disorders in humanitarian settings need to be accompanied by studies that validate the tool used to diagnose the disorders. Validating the tool ensures that there is a meaningful distinction between mental disorders and non-pathological psychological distress (see also IASC, 2007, page 45).[6]

If you have to make a quick estimate on the prevalence of mental disorders, you can use existing WHO projections for a general indication of mental disorders in crisis-affected populations (see below in Table 3.2). However, you should acknowledge that this is only an estimate and that observed rates vary widely depending on the context and method of study.

---

[4] All of the HESPER items (see Tool 3) measure people's *subjective* experience and are thereby psychosocial in nature.
[5] The *Multi-cluster/sector Initial Rapid Assessment* (MIRA) approach (which is currently being developed) aims to be the standard intersectoral tool used by IASC Clusters for assessment of the humanitarian situation in the first two weeks after a major sudden-onset emergency.
[6] For more on this issue, see Bolton & Betancourt, 2004, Horwith, 2007, Rodin & van Ommeren, 2009.

In general, it is important to note the following:
- Both (a) adversity (loss and potentially traumatic events) and (b) an insecure, unsupportive recovery environment are associated with higher rates of mental disorder (Steel et al, 2009).
- Higher-quality studies (involving diagnostic tools, random samples and large sample sizes) are associated with lower rates of mental disorder (Steel et al, 2009).[7]
- Studies that do not take into account assessment of clinical significance or impaired functioning identify much higher rates of disorders (Breslau et al, 2007). This is generally the case for most studies involving self-report measures.

Although the toolkit does not cover measuring mental disorders, it does cover surveys of serious mental health symptoms. Agencies are often interested in knowing, monitoring and reporting on such problems in a population, and this may be done relatively quickly without assessing mental disorders (see Tool 2). Experience with Tool 2 has shown that you can effectively use such surveys for making a case (advocacy) for more attention to mental health in humanitarian settings.

TABLE 3.2	WHO PROJECTIONS OF MENTAL DISORDERS IN ADULT POPULATIONS AFFECTED BY EMERGENCIES[i]	
	Before the emergency: 12-month prevalence (median across countries and across level of exposure to adversity)[ii]	After the emergency: 12-month prevalence (median across countries and across level of exposure to adversity)
Severe disorder (for example, psychosis, severe depression, severely disabling form of anxiety disorder)	2% to 3%	3% to 4%[iii]
Mild or moderate mental disorder (for example, mild and moderate forms of depression and anxiety disorders, including mild and moderate PTSD)	10%	15% to 20%[iv]
Normal distress / other psychological reactions (no disorder)	No estimate	Large percentage

Notes: Adapted from WHO (2005). PTSD indicates post-traumatic stress disorder.
[i] Observed rates vary with setting (for example, time since the emergency, socio-cultural factors in coping and community social support, previous and current disaster exposure) and the assessment method.
[ii] The assumed baseline rates are the median rates across countries as observed in the World Mental Health Survey 2000.
[iii] This is a best guess based on the assumption that traumatic events and loss may contribute to a relapse in previously stable mental disorders, and also may cause severely disabling forms of mood and anxiety disorders.
[iv] It is established that traumatic events and loss increase the risk of depression and anxiety disorders, including posttraumatic stress disorder.

---

7   Steel et al's (2009) meta-analysis of the more robust epidemiological surveys (those using random samples and diagnostic interviews) among populations affected by conflict has found average prevalence rates of 15.4% (30 studies) and 17.3 % (26 studies) for post-traumatic stress disorder (PTSD) and depression respectively. These rates are substantially higher than the average prevalence of 7.6% (any anxiety disorder, including PTSD) and 5.3% (any mood disorder, including major depressive disorder) observed across 17 national representative samples participating in the World Mental Health Survey.

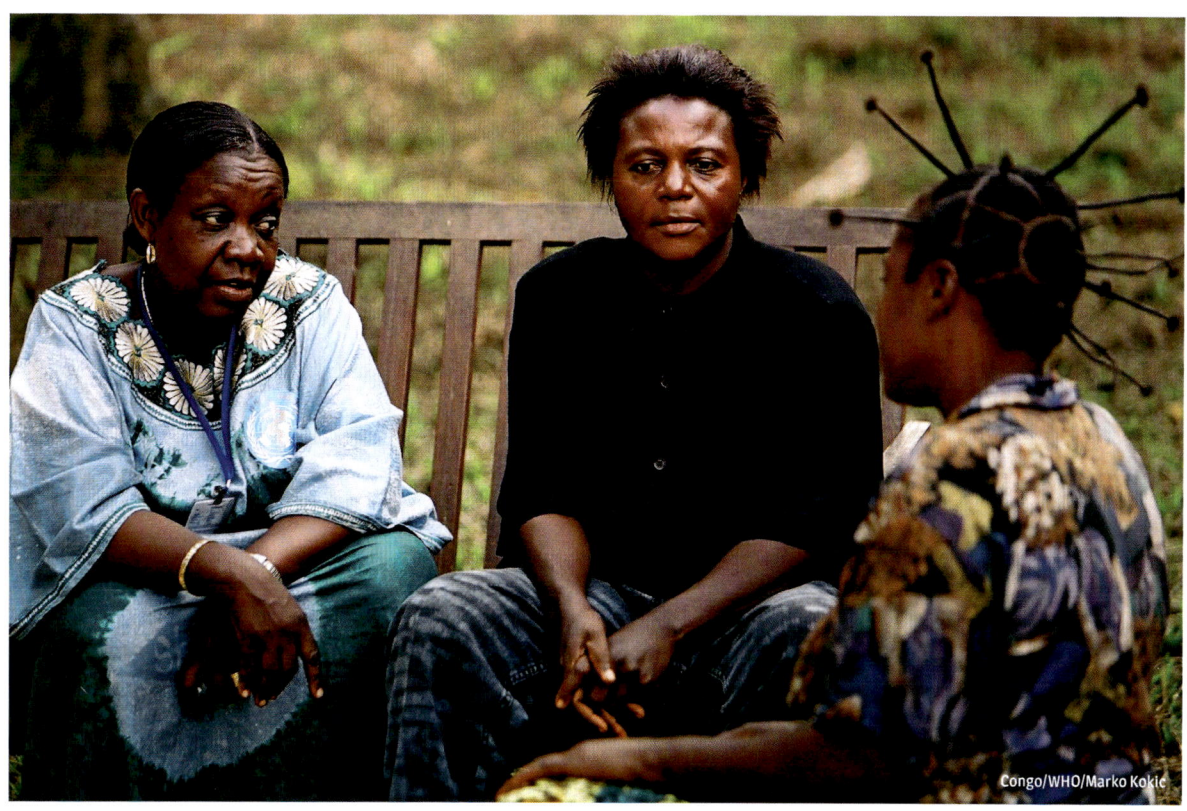

3.3. COLLECTING QUALITATIVE AND QUANTITATIVE DATA

3.3.1 General guidance on collecting qualitative and quantitative data

General guidance on collecting qualitative and quantitative data is given below.

1. Informed consent: Assessments present a significant burden for those taking part. They take up important time and energy and may remind people of hardship, often in situations that are already challenging. It is very important that participants only join assessments on a voluntary basis and understand what you expect of them. In a humanitarian crisis this is often more difficult, because assessors often represent agencies that provide assistance. People may join assessments because they expect assistance from these agencies. It is important that you are completely honest with potential participants; if you are not sure whether assessment will be linked to action, you should make this clear. Such honesty includes keeping any promises you make for assistance. False promises undermine community participation and effective humanitarian assistance.

> **Further reading**
>
> World Health Organization (2003). WHO Ethical and Safety Recommendations for Interviewing Trafficked Women. Geneva: WHO
> http://www.who.int/gender/documents/en/final%20recommendations%2023%20oct.pdf

2. Interview setting: Where you conduct an interview can have a big influence on the results. You should, as far as possible, make sure that participants feel free to speak without being watched, interrupted by others, reminded of things they need to do, and so on. It is important to think through the logistics of where you will hold interviews, **before** the assessment team goes into specific assessment locations.

3. Language: Participants may discuss mental health and psychosocial problems in many ways. Mental disorders can easily be confused with normal distress, that is, being unhappy or upset. Local languages may or may not have words for this distinction (for example in Nepali a distinction is made between the heart-mind *man* and brain-mind *dimaag*, with problems in the *man* being less stigmatised). The same word may mean something different in different cultures. For example the word 'bored' in English refers to 'frustration' in some South Asian communities, and the word *traumatized* can have different meaning in different cultures. Also, different cultures will have different ways of distinguishing mental health problems from other problems. For example, problems that you may think are interesting from a mental health point of view, may be experienced as supernatural problems by participants (for example hearing voices from evil spirits or fainting attacks). Sometimes lay language for mental disorders is stigmatising (for example, in English 'crazy' or 'has a screw loose'). You should choose words with great care so as not to stigmatise participants. It is crucial that you translate technical terms in any interviewing tools carefully, informed by the desk review or preliminary key informant interviews.

4. Attitude: An important aspect of interviewing rests in the way that the interviewer approaches participants, and is able to form a relationship of trust and rapport. This topic should be included in the training of the assessment team, for example through a brainstorm with all team members on essential characteristics for sensitive interviewing. These may include:
- attitudes, for example: willingness to listen; openness towards other opinions; being non-judgemental; curiosity; flexibility; willingness to travel and work in different places at irregular times; and
- skills, for example; active listening; ability to create an atmosphere of confidence; note-taking skills; ability to follow interviewing instructions; gaining interviewing experience through role play; and ability to think of alternative strategies if unexpected situations come up.

> **Further reading**
> Hardon, A. (2001). Applied Health Research. Amsterdam: het Spinhuis.
> http://openlibrary.org/books/OL9106217M/Applied_Health_Research-Manual

5. Bias: Bias refers to a systematic influence on the information that was not intended. For example, people may answer questions about how they are doing with strongly negative answers because they think this may help for them to get access to services. Or, people may not describe any negative emotions because they do not want to appear weak in the eyes of others. In addition, interviewers may be biased, which may influence responses. It is important that assessment teams reflect and report on how answers to questions may be biased.

6. Recording verbatim data: Many of the tools in this toolbox ask for specific information that can be recorded verbatim (that is, *literally*, as the words were spoken) on paper. Ideally, qualitative data is collected verbatim, and in most interview situations you can use tape recorders for this purpose. However, in humanitarian settings using a tape recorder may lead to security concerns or is often just not feasible or appropriate. In situations where rapid information collection and analysis are crucial (for example phase 1 to 3), good note taking may be a good alternative to tape-recording.

7. Storing data: The information that you collect during an assessment (for example tape-recorded data, interview transcripts) provides the basis for recommendations for action and represents significant efforts and sacrifices by participants. So you should treat data with the utmost care and respect. You should take care that data:
- remains safe and secure (for example, from army personnel or camp leadership);
- is kept clean (for example in plastic sheets to protect it from humidity, food, dirt);
- is systematically kept (for example in numbered boxes); and
- is made anonymous to protect confidentiality. To achieve anonymity, the forms with data should only contain participant numbers, while you keep a list with corresponding names and numbers securely locked under the responsibility of the team leader.

3.3.2 Qualitative assessments

Some of the tools in this toolbox concern collecting qualitative data, within a rapid appraisal format. The next sections are intended as a very short primer on the topic of collecting qualitative data. You can find more information in 'further reading' boxes.

3.3.2.1 Key informant interviews

Key informant interviews (a technique used in Tools 1, 4, 5, 9, 10, 11 and 12) are interviews with people that are considered to be in a good position to provide the information you need. For instance, if you are interested in local mourning rituals, you may consider religious leaders as key informants. Key informant interviews often involve repeated open-ended interviews with the same person.

There are a number of strengths associated with using key informant interviews, including:
- the possibility of examining topics in-depth by asking key informants to clarify information or explanations a number of times in a flexible manner;
- key informants may provide relatively easy access to a wealth of knowledge; and
- key informants often enjoy sharing their knowledge.

A limitation of using key informants is that information comes from a relatively small, select group of individuals. Also, you cannot assume that people who you select as key informants will actually have accurate knowledge of the issues you are assessing. It is not always easy to evaluate whether the opinions of these individuals are representative of the complete group of people that you are assessing. Also, interviewing key informants requires good interviewing skills, which might not always be readily available. One important limitation of using key informant interviews in emergencies is that analysing narrative data requires substantial skill and time.

> **Further reading**
> - IASC (2012). Annex IV Key informant interviews. In The Multi Cluster/Sector Initial Rapid Assessment (MIRA) (provisional version) IASC. ochanet.unocha.org/p/Documents/mira_final_version2012.pdf
> - Center for Substance Abuse Prevention's Northeast Center for the Application of Prevention Technologies (2004). Data Collection Methods: Getting Down to Basics: Key Informant Interviews. New York: Education Development Center http://www.oasas.ny.gov/prevention/needs/documents/KeyInformantInterviews.pdf
> - Kumar, K. (1989) Conducting Key Informant Interviews in Developing Countries. Agency for International Development/. http://pdf.usaid.gov/pdf_docs/pnaax226.pdf
> - Varkevisser, C.M., Pathmanathan, I., Brownlee, A. (2003). Developing and Conducting Health Systems Research Projects. Volume II: Data Analysis and Report Writing. Amsterdam: KIT Publishers/ IDRC/ WHO AFRO http://www.kit.nl/net/KIT_Publicaties_output/ShowFile2.aspx?e=587

3.3.2.2 Group interviews

Group interviews (a technique used in Tool 11) are meetings in which participants (often selected because they are similar in age, gender, profession, social status and so on) are asked to answer questions. When participants are encouraged to react to each other's comments and to expand each other's answers, they are called focus group interviews.

Group interviews are a good way to identify community opinions on issues and the different views held by different sub-groups. They are also useful to reach a larger number of people at the same time and to begin to identify the local language that people use to discuss things. The group is not expected to produce a consensus, as the assessors are looking for all points of view on a topic.

One of the main risks in group interviews is that a few people in the group may dominate the discussion (for example those with higher social standing), thus obscuring the different views of group members. When conducting group interviews it is important to:
- limit the group size to 8 to 12 participants; and
- keep group members as homogeneous (similar) as possible, especially regarding age and gender, so people are more likely have the confidence to actively take part.

Also, the facilitation of a good group interview requires training on probing and group facilitation skills. In general, two people conduct group interviews with one person asking questions and steering the discussion, while the other person takes notes.

Group interviews are generally not appropriate for questions on very sensitive topics, when people may feel uncomfortable responding honestly in the presence of others. Finally, because different groups may have different answers to questions, you need to organise at least two group interviews for each topic to make sure you hear all opinions (saturation).

> **Further reading**
> - Heary, C.M. & Hennessy, E. (2002). The use of focus groups in pediatric health research. Journal of Pediatric Psychology, 27, 47-57. http://jpepsy.oxfordjournals.org/cgi/content/full/27/1/47
> - Wong, L.P. (2008). Focus Group Discussion: a tool for health and medical research. Singapore Medical Journal, 49, 256-260. http://smj.sma.org.sg/4903/4903me1.pdf

3.3.2.3 Free listing

Free listing (a technique used in Tools 10 and 12) involves asking an individual (often a general community member) to provide as many answers to a single question as possible. For instance, you can ask people to list the types of problems they have or the kind of coping methods they use. You can follow free listing by asking participants to prioritise or categorise their answers. From a free list, you can choose problems (for example, mental health and psychosocial problems) for further assessment through other types of assessment methods (for example individual or group interviews). Generally, it is easier to ask participants to discuss the experiences of others (for example about general members of their community) than their own experiences, especially in group settings. Free listing is often useful at the beginning of an assessment to get an overview of the types of problems and resources in a community.

Participative ranking (Ager, Stark & Potts, 2009) is similar to free listing. Participants are asked, generally in a group format, what types of problems they feel are present in a humanitarian setting. Then, participants are asked to identify objects to represent those problems (for example, a beer glass for alcohol use, a stone for domestic violence). Then, all the objects are placed in a line in order of importance (ranking). The whole process can then be repeated for resources (for example a book for supportive teachers, a tree branch for women groups). This method may have advantages when assessing relatively abstract concepts such as mental health and psychosocial problems.

The main advantage of free listing techniques is that they are relatively quick ways of collecting information on specific issues, and they can be done with a variety of informants (for example youth, men, women, people with disabilities). Also, results are much quicker and easier to analyse and compile compared with narrative data collected through open-ended questions from key informant interviews or focus groups. The disadvantages with these methods are that they generally provide less detailed information on the context. Another disadvantage is that these techniques depend highly on the exact phrasing of the question, which increases the risk of missing out on important information. Also, when you apply these techniques in a group, respondents may bias their responses towards what the other group members may want to hear. Nonetheless, these techniques are useful in acute emergencies, because they are able to provide valuable information in a very short time span.

Further reading

- Ager, A, Stark, L & Potts, A (2009) Participative Ranking Methodology: A Brief Guide (Version 1.1, February 2010). Program on Forced Migration & Health, Mailman School of Public Health, Columbia University, New York.
- Public Health Action Support Team (2010). Qualitative methods. In Public Health Action Support Team. Public Health Textbook. London: Public Health Action Support Team http://www.healthknowledge.org.uk/public-health-textbook/research-methods/1d-qualitative-methods
- Applied Mental Health Research Group. (forthcoming). *Design, implementation, monitoring, and evaluation of cross-cultural mental health and psychosocial assistance programs: a user's manual for researchers and program implementers*. Baltimore: Center for Refugee and Disaster Response, Johns Hopkins University School of Public Health

3.3.2.4 Deciding on the number of participants in qualitative assessments

When carrying out qualitative assessments, you would mostly collect data until 'data saturation' takes place. Data saturation has occurred when the same responses are provided repeatedly. For instance, after fourteen semi-structured interviews, the last two or three interviews might not provide any new or different answers. When using qualitative techniques it is usually not possible to determine beforehand how many people are needed. In practice, however, planning and budgeting are difficult without an estimate of the number of interviews you are going to conduct. We have provided these estimates in the introduction to the tools.

3.3.2.5 Analysing qualitative data

When collecting qualitative data, it is generally useful to do a preliminary data analysis while the collection is ongoing (for example, at the end of each data collection session). It can help to establish preliminary ideas and tighten the data collection plan accordingly (for example, filling gaps in knowledge on specific groups of participants, or changing the type of questions). Assessment team leaders should analyse at least some data while it is collected, to monitor the quality of data collection and the nature of the data as it comes in. This may best be done through daily meetings with the assessment team or by routinely technically debriefing local interviewers as they return from interviews. These meetings should also function to monitor the wellbeing of assessment staff working in challenging circumstances. During these meetings, general themes arising from interviews may be discussed, and the data collection plans revised accordingly.

There are a variety of ways to analyse qualitative data. These range from sophisticated, time-consuming analyses aimed at constructing theories about social phenomena to simply grouping answers together and labelling them. For humanitarian purposes, grouping answers together and labelling them is often appropriate. For example the analyst reads the text and identifies themes. They then reread all responses to categorise text that relate to the themes. Ideally this is done by two independent analysts who compare results to reduce the risk of bias.

With regard to triangulation, it may happen that data from different sources on the same subject are inconsistent. Any such inconsistencies should be reported and discussed.

4. Translating assessment into action

4.1 DRAFTING A REPORT WITH RECOMMENDATIONS

The main goal of an assessment is to provide recommendations for action. Generally, the more precise a recommendation, the more useful it is.

Recommendations for humanitarian activities should specify:
- who you are making the recommendation to;
- the target group;
- the problem targeted;
- the suggested intervention, or how the intervention may be developed together with the target population; and
- links with relevant guidance (for example specifying an action sheet from the IASC MHPSS guidelines).

When there are a number of recommendations, you should put them in order of priority. The report should communicate that actions should be carried out following rank order of priorities.

The report should be clear which recommendations are short term (that is, should be put in place immediately) and which recommendations are longer term. As far as possible you should discuss ideas for recommendations with the target group before you put them on paper.

The IASC MHPSS guidelines recommend providing MHPSS in a multi-layered system of care. It can often be helpful to cross reference recommendations with the four layers of the IASC pyramid (for an example, see the Healthnet TPO (2009) assessment report on Afghanistan).

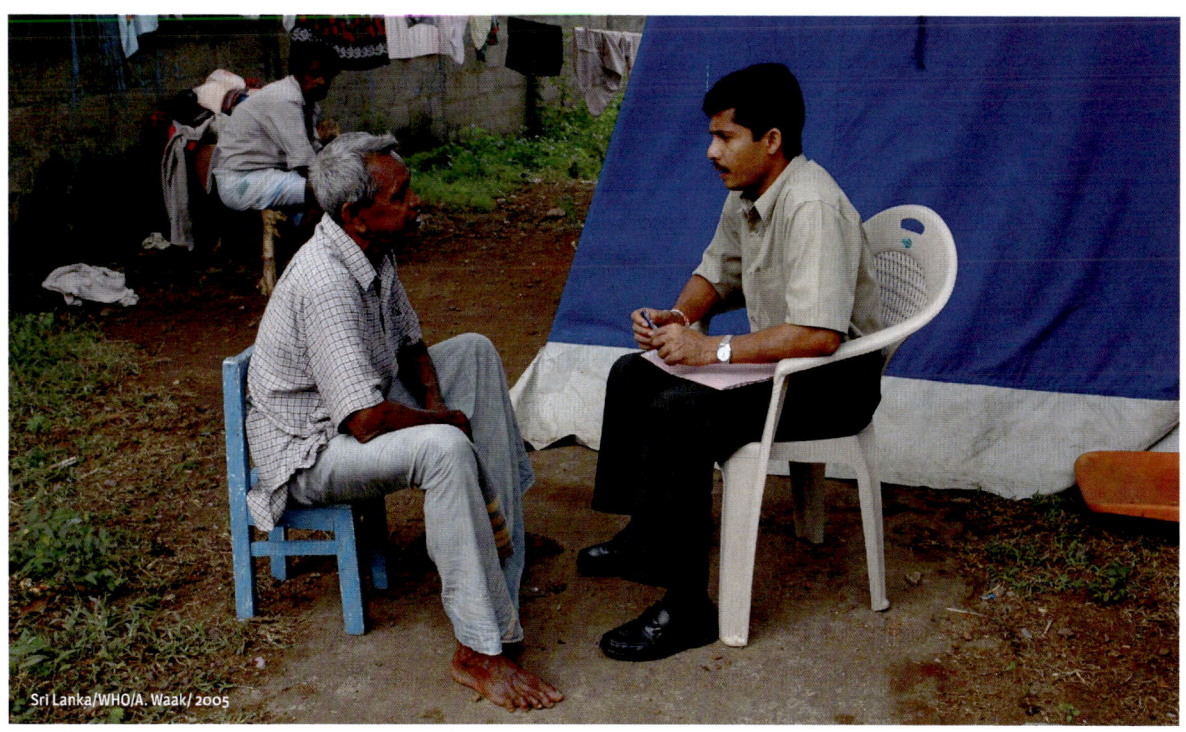
Sri Lanka/WHO/A. Waak/ 2005

FIGURE 4.1   THE IASC PYRAMID (ADAPTED WITH PERMISSION)

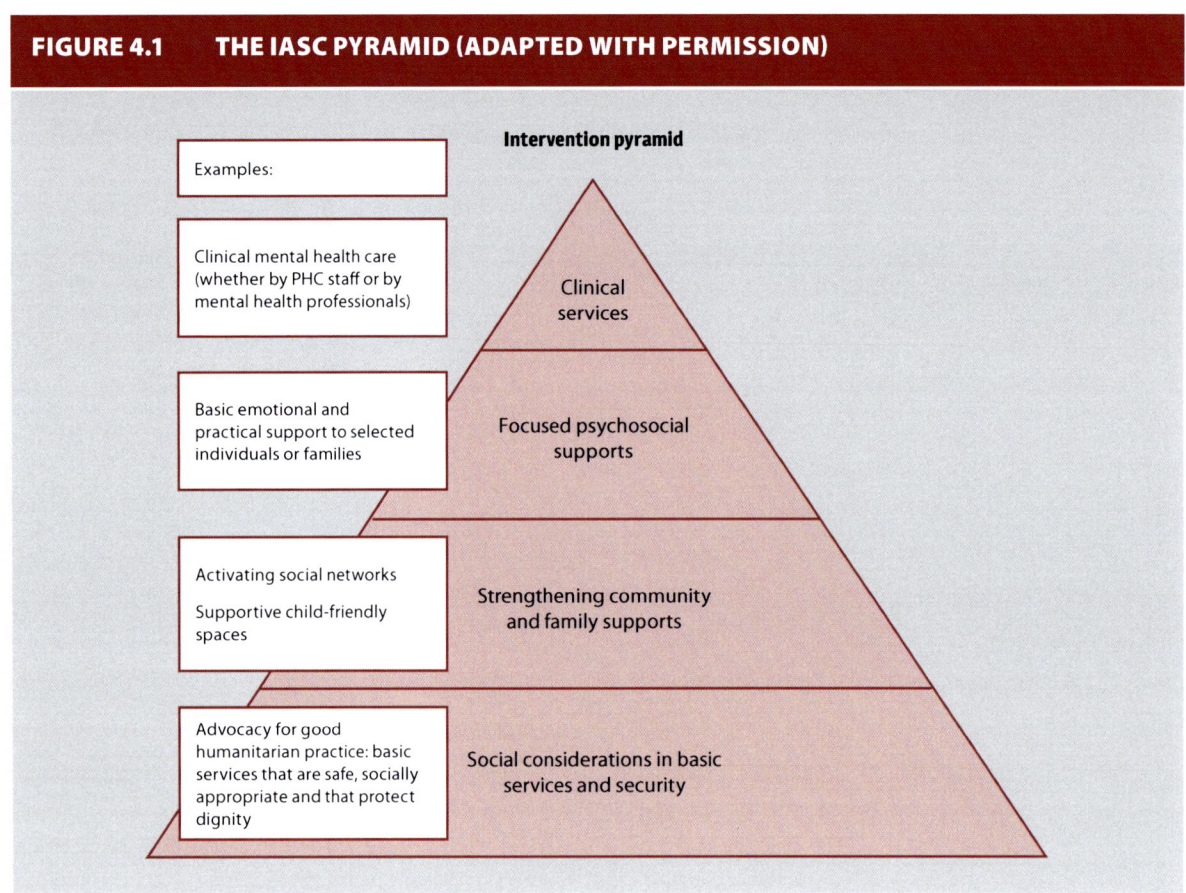

4.2 COMMUNICATING RECOMMENDATIONS

To make the most of any assessment, you should share recommendations with all relevant stakeholders. These include the government, the people you are targeting with the programs, and local communities, and other humanitarian and health actors. If you don't feed assessment information back to communities, you may possibly leave affected people feeling exploited. You can share recommendations with stakeholders by organising meetings to discuss the key findings.

All assessment reports should include a summary in plain lay language to ensure that stakeholders can understand key findings along with the assessment's limitations and recommendations. Where possible, you should accompany the assessment with a short power point presentation of this plain-language summary.

Sharing the assessment report with relevant stakeholders is crucial to implementing humanitarian action in line with the best available information – maximising the positive impact of action while lowering the risk of unintentional harm.

So, agencies should put their findings in the public domain and consider the following points.

1. **Security risks**. Security risks can occur when the assessment report identifies information that may put people at risk of harm. This situation is more likely to occur in assessments focusing on protection issues. For example, during interviews with key informants, participants may report information on human rights violations against their religious or ethnic group. In such situations, you should report the information to relevant trust-worthy protection bodies and you should not include it in the overall public reporting.

2. **Agency competition**. Agency competition for funding must **not** prevent dissemination of the main results and recommendations. Agencies should be able to use each others' assessment reports, and they should do this with proper acknowledgement of the agency that collected the information.

3. **Sensitive information.** An assessment may show that national or international agencies are delivering poor services and support. Whether it is appropriate to put such information in the public domain will depend on the situation. In any case, you should make all efforts to communicate the information in a constructive manner to the relevant agency. You should put all other findings of the assessment in the overall MHPSS needs assessment report which should go in the public domain.

4. **Academic publication**. Academic journals occasionally do not allow the publication of assessment reports that have already been disseminated widely (for example by posting on a website). However, this is **not** an acceptable reason to postpone disseminating at least a plain-language version of the report with the main results and recommendations.

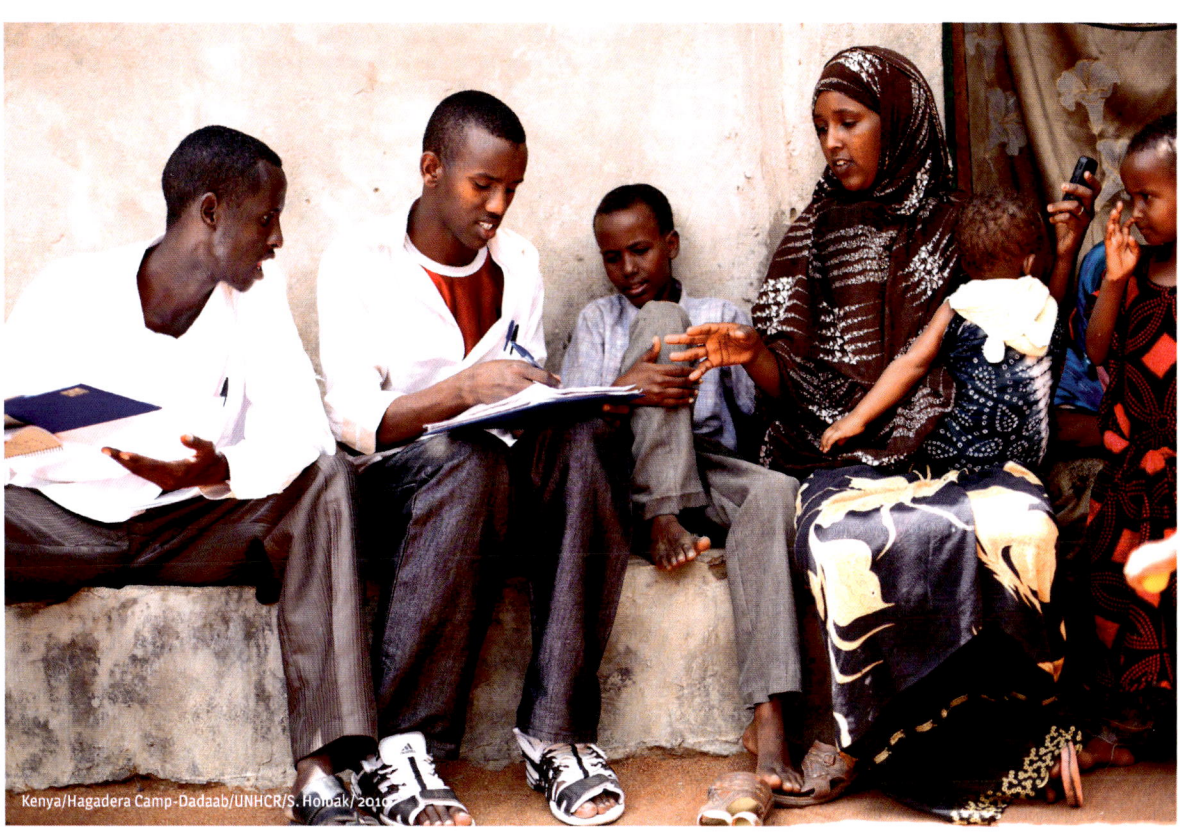

Kenya/Hagadera Camp-Dadaab/UNHCR/S. Hopak/2010

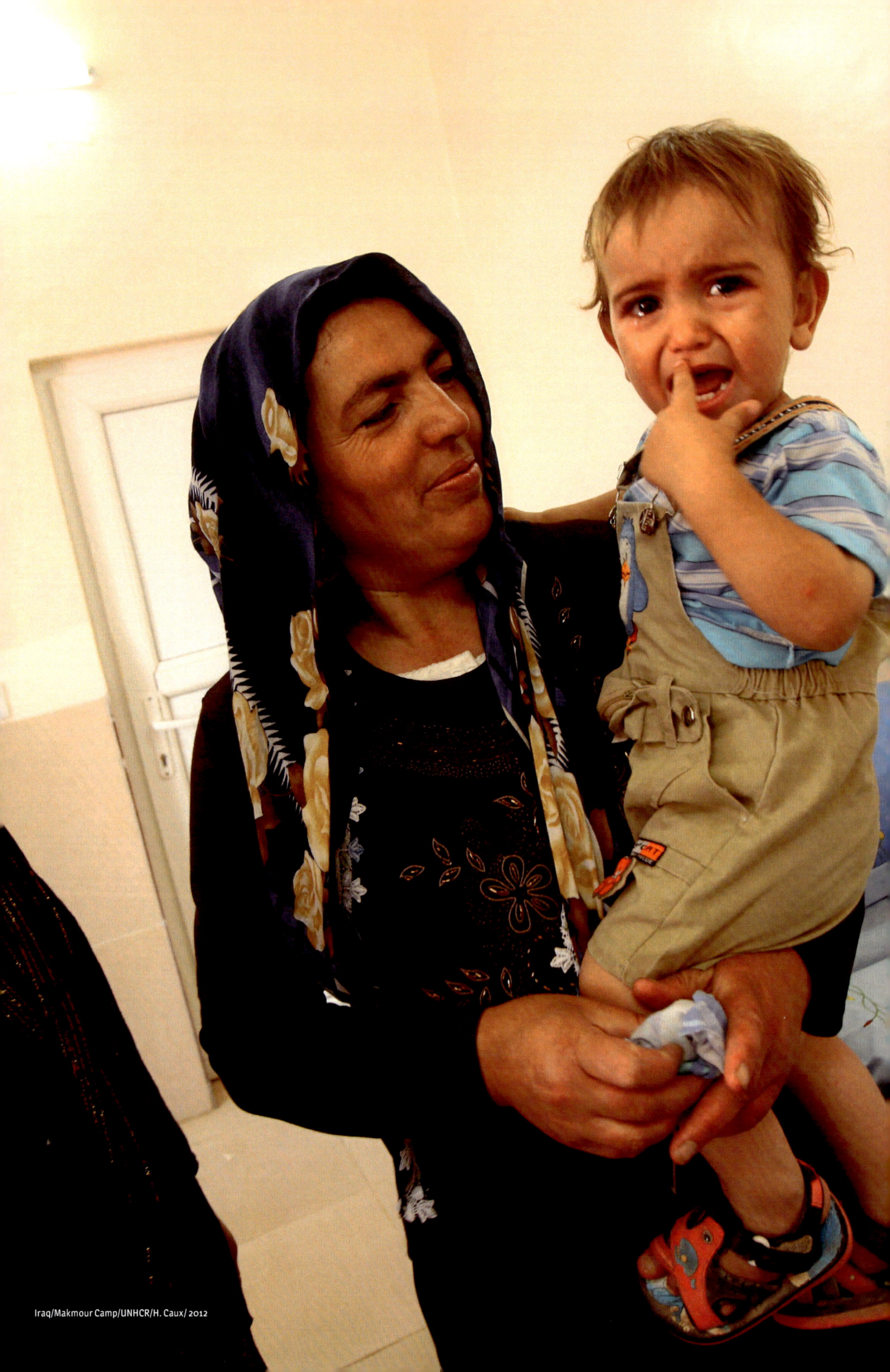
Iraq/Makmour Camp/UNHCR/H. Caux/ 2012

ASSESSMENT TOOLS

TOOL 1 — WHO IS WHERE, WHEN, DOING WHAT (4WS) IN MENTAL HEALTH AND PSYCHOSOCIAL SUPPORT: SUMMARY OF MANUAL WITH ACTIVITY CODES[8]

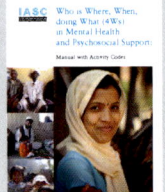

Why use this tool: For coordination, through mapping what mental health and psychosocial supports are available

Method: Interviews with agency programme managers

Time needed: Depending on the scale of the crisis, approximately two weeks initially (needs regular updating)

Human resources needed: Two people

Background

- A Who is Where, When, doing What (4Ws) tool for MHPSS is useful for the following:
    - (a) Providing a big picture of the size and nature of the response.
    - (b) Identifying gaps in the response to enable coordinated action.
    - (c) Enabling referral by making information available about who is where doing what.
    - (d) Informing appeal processes (for example, the Consolidated Appeal Process, CAP).
    - (e) Improving transparency and legitimacy of MHPSS through structured documentation.
    - (f) Improving possibilities for reviewing patterns of practice and for drawing lessons for future response.

- This 4Ws tool is a software-based data system to map MHPSS activities in humanitarian settings across sectors.

- In many situations it may not be feasible for individuals to successfully collect the data. Collecting data from different agencies requires leverage and is best done by agencies (government, UN or NGOs) with coordination responsibilities.

- Data is collected through an Excel spreadsheet. The file needs to be completed by each organisation participating in the 4W exercise. The items to be completed for this sheet can be found in Table 1. This sheet refers to MHPSS activity codes displayed in Table 2.

- The relationship between the activity codes in Table 2 and the Action Sheets and Pyramid of the IASC Guidelines is described in an annex of the manual that comes with the 4Ws tool.

- You should read the whole manual carefully before using the tool. The manual describes suggested steps to implement the 4Ws tool for MHPSS including:
    - (a) translating and adapting the 4Ws data collection spreadsheet for the local context;
    - (b) contacting the government or the UN coordinating agency to obtain standard spelling and codes of geographical areas, specifying the boundaries of geographical areas;
    - (c) deciding on the scope and strategy for data collection;
    - (d) approaching agencies, collecting data and reviewing collected data;
    - (e) reviewing collected data for major inconsistencies or errors, cleaning-up and merging data;
    - (f) analysing data and preparing and disseminating a report on the results;
    - (g) discussing identified gaps with stakeholders and deciding on improved programming; and
    - (h) updating the data and reports.

---

8   Source: IASC Reference Group on Mental Health and Psychosocial Support in Emergency Settings. Who is Where, When, doing What (4Ws) in Mental Health and Psychosocial Support: Manual with Activity Codes (Field Test Version). Geneva: 2012. This tool has been reproduced here in summary form with permission from the IASC Reference Group. http://www.who.int/mental_health/publications/iasc_4ws/en/index.html

- As mentioned, this 4Ws tool maps MHPSS across sectors. However, if you are interested only in mapping MHPSS within a specific sector, you should use a 4Ws tool that is sector specific. The 4Ws tool of the global health cluster is the IASC Global Health Cluster's (2009) *Health Resources Availability Mapping (HeRAMS) system*.
  (a) HeRAMS should be implemented by or under the health sector leadership (for example Ministry of Health, Health Cluster).
  (b) HeRAMS provides a health services checklist by level of care, by health sub-sectors, and for health facility/mobile clinic/community-based interventions at each point of delivery. There are specific mental health checklist items under the community care, primary care and secondary and tertiary care levels.
  (c) People who organize mental health assessments are usually not in the position to initiate HeRAMS. However, wherever HeRAMS is implemented, they should ensure that mental health services are recorded in HeRAMS, and use HeRAMS as a key source of relevant mental health services information.

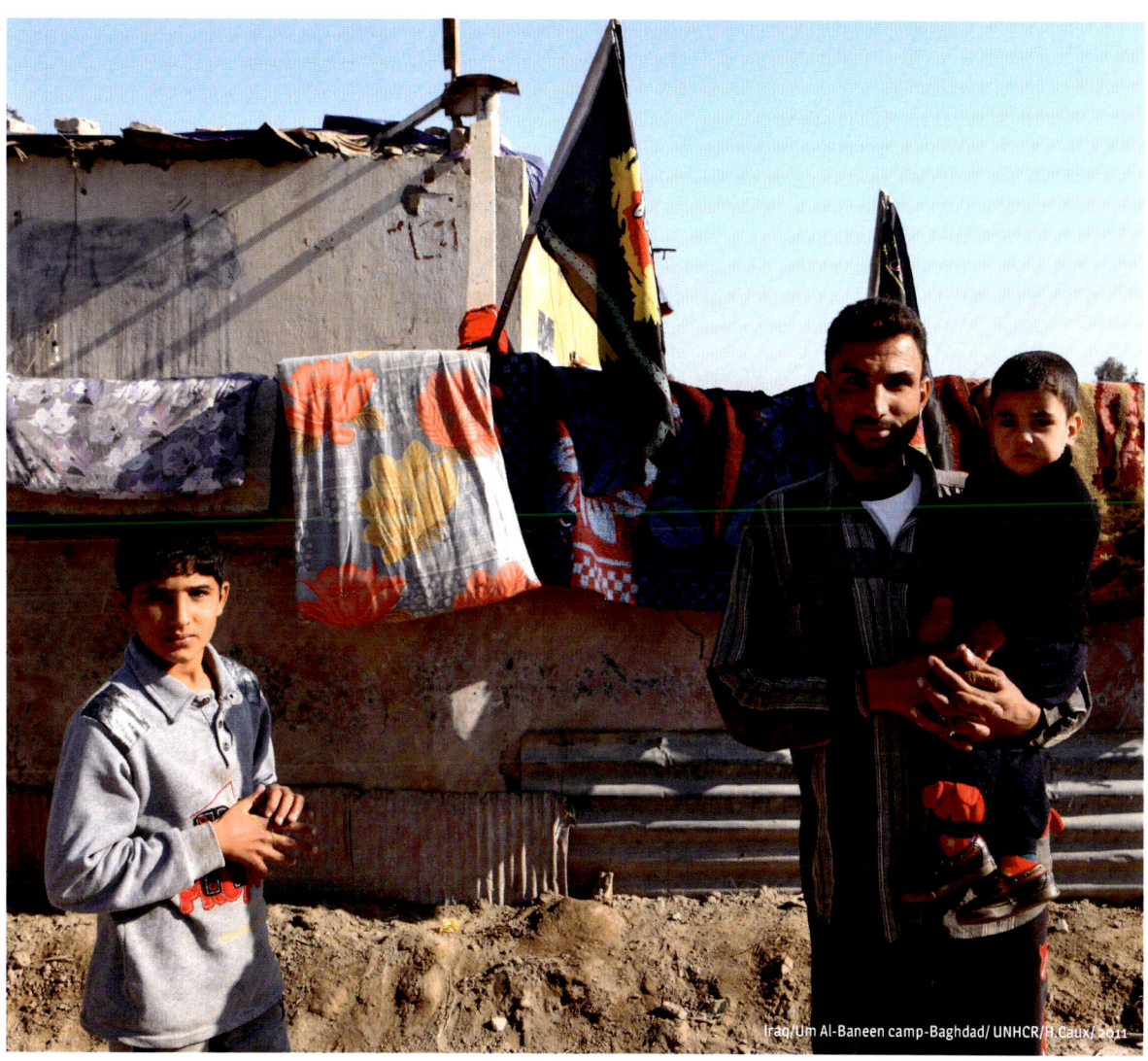

Iraq/Um Al-Baneen camp-Baghdad/ UNHCR/H.Caux/ 2011

TABLE 1 OF TOOL 1: ITEMS TO BE COMPLETED IN THE SECOND SHEET OF THE 4WS DATA COLLECTION SPREADSHEET

A. Date of providing or updating this information
B. Name of implementing agency
C. Name(s) of other organization(s) with whom this activity is done (in case of a joint activity)
D. Name of the focal point
E. Phone number of the focal point
F. Email address of the focal point
G. Region / district where the activity occurs
H. Town/ neighbourhood where the activity occurs
I. Government/ OCHA geographical code for the location
J. MHPSS activity code
K. MHPSS activity subcode
L. Description of the activity in one sentence (for subcode "Other" or for any other activity that is not clearly described by the subcode)
M. Target group(s) (specify age group(s) where relevant)
N. Number of people in target group directly supported in previous 30 days
O. This activity is (1) currently being implemented, (2) funded but not yet implemented, or (3) unfunded and not yet implemented
P. Start date for implementing the activity (for current activities, provide actual start date and not the originally proposed start date)
Q. End date (specify on what date committed funding to implement the activity ends)

Optional (The following 5 optional items give a better understanding of possible quality and volume of the services available but: may be too detailed for the first weeks or months of an acute major crisis.)

R. Number and type of MHPSS workers who do this activity (e.g., 4 community volunteers, 1 psychologist and 1 nurse)
S. Topic and length of non-university training on MHPSS (e.g. nurses received 1 day on psychological first aid)
T. (if applicable) Availability of the activity (e.g. child friendly space or clinic is open 40 hours/week)
U. Where is MHPSS provided? (people's homes, clinic, public spaces etc.)
V. Do people have to pay to use these services/supports?

TABLE 2 OF TOOL 1. MHPSS ACTIVITY CODES AND SUBCODES

READ THIS FIRST!
- MHPSS stands for mental health and psychosocial support.
- The list includes the most common activities that are conducted under the heading of MHPSS in large humanitarian crises.
- The list is not exhaustive. You should use the category 'other (describe in column C of the data entry sheet)' to document activities not included in the list.
- The list is descriptive rather than prescriptive. No judgement is passed whether included activities are appropriate or not. A number of the mentioned activities are or can be controversial. For guidance on recommended practices, see IASC (2007).
- **INSTRUCTION: FILL IN THE RELEVANT MHPSS ACTIVITY CODE (SEE COLUMN A BELOW) AND SUBCODE (SEE COLUMN B BELOW) IN COLUMNS A AND B OF THE DATA ENTRY SHEET. IF ONE WORKS BROADLY IN AN AREA, THEN CHOOSE THE SUBCODE 'OTHER'.**

	Column A: MHPSS activity code (4Ws)	Column B: Examples of interventions with subcodes. Record all that apply.
Community-focussed (targeted at communities or segments of communities)	1. Disseminating information to the community at large	1.1 Information on the current situation, relief efforts or available services in general 1.2 Raising awareness on mental health and psychosocial support (e.g., messages on positive coping or on available mental health services and psychosocial supports) 1.3 Other (describe in column C of the data entry sheet)
	2. Facilitating conditions for community mobilisation, community organisation, community ownership or community control over emergency relief in general	2.1 Support for emergency relief that is initiated by the community 2.2 Support for communal spaces/meetings to discuss, problem-solve and plan action by community members to respond to the emergency 2.3 Other (describe in column C of the data entry sheet)
	3. Strengthening community and family support	3.1 Support for social support activities that are initiated by the community 3.2 Strengthening parenting/family supports 3.3 Facilitation of community supports to vulnerable people 3.4 Structured social activities (e.g. group activities) 3.5 Structured recreational or creative activities (do not include activities at child-friendly spaces that are covered in 4.1) 3.6 Early childhood development (ECD) activities 3.7 Facilitation of conditions for indigenous traditional, spiritual or religious supports, including communal healing practices 3.8 Other (describe in column C of the data entry sheet)
	4. Safe spaces	4.1 Child-friendly spaces 4.2 Other (describe in column C of the data entry sheet)
	5. Psychosocial support in education	5.1 Psychosocial support to teachers / other personnel at schools/learning places 5.2 Psychosocial support to classes/groups of children at schools/learning places 5.3 Other (describe in column C of the data entry sheet)
	6. Supporting including social/psychosocial considerations in protection, health services, nutrition, food aid, shelter, site planning or water and sanitation	6.1 Orientation of or advocacy with aid workers/agencies on including social/ psychosocial considerations in programming (specify sector in column C of the data entry sheet) 6.2 Other (describe in column C of the data entry sheet)
Person-focused (targeted at identified people)	7. (Person-focused) psychosocial work	7.1 Psychological first aid (PFA) 7.2 Linking vulnerable individuals/families to resources (e.g., health services, livelihoods assistance, community resources etc.) and following up to see if support is provided. 7.3 Other (describe in column C of the data entry sheet)
	8. Psychological intervention	8.1 Basic counselling for individuals (specify type in column C of the data entry sheet) 8.2 Basic counselling for groups or families (specify type in column C of the data entry sheet) 8.3 Interventions for alcohol/substance use problems (specify type in column C of the data entry sheet) 8.4 Psychotherapy (specify type in column C of the data entry sheet) 8.5 Individual or group psychological debriefing 8.6 Other (describe in column C of the data entry sheet)
	9. Clinical management of mental disorders by nonspecialized health care providers (eg PHC, post-surgery wards)	9.1 Non-pharmacological management of mental disorder by nonspecialized health care providers (where possible specify type of support using categories 7 and 8) 9.2 Pharmacological management of mental disorder by nonspecialized health care providers 9.3 Action by community workers to identify and refer people with mental disorders and to follow-up on them to make sure adherence to clinical treatment 9.4 Other (describe in column C of the data entry sheet)
	10. Clinical management of mental disorders by specialized mental health care providers (eg psychiatrists, psychiatric nurses and psychologists working at PHC/general health facilities/mental health facilities)	10.1 Non-pharmacological management of mental disorder by specialized mental health care providers (where possible specify type of support using categories 7 and 8) 10.2 Pharmacological management of mental disorder by specialized health care 10.3 Inpatient mental health care 10.4 Other (describe in column C of the data entry sheet)
General	11. General activities to support MHPSS	11.1 Situation analyses/assessment 11.2 Monitoring/evaluation 11.3 Training / orienting (specify topic in column C of the data entry sheet) 11.4 Technical or clinical supervision 11.5 Psychosocial support for aid workers (describe type in column C of the data entry sheet) 11.6 Research 11.7 Other (describe in column C of the data entry sheet)

TOOL 2	WHO-UNHCR ASSESSMENT SCHEDULE OF SERIOUS SYMPTOMS IN HUMANITARIAN SETTINGS (WASSS) (FIELD-TEST VERSION)[9]

Why use this tool: For advocacy, by showing the prevalence of mental health problems in the community

Method: Part of a community household survey (representative sample)

Time needed: Two to three minutes for each interview covering part A of this tool, and five minutes for each interview covering part B

Human resources needed: interviewers, one analyst/report-writer

Background

Health surveys and surveillance in humanitarian crisis settings offer the opportunity to assess how common mental health problems are in the affected population. This short tool contains mental health questions that you could consider adding to general health surveys and surveillance in humanitarian crises. The tool is meant to be applied by humanitarian health actors and can be administered by lay interviewers without specific mental health expertise.

The purpose of this tool is to identify persons in priority need of mental health care. So, the selected questions are meant to identify people with symptoms of severe distress and impaired functioning.

It is useful to identify these people:

- to describe to public health decision-makers the extent to which specific mental health problems are an issue (advocacy); and
- to potentially inform community mental health services whether an interviewee potentially has a mental disorder (screening).

The tool does *not* assess rates of mental disorders. Both mental disorders and transient (temporary) stress reactions are more likely to occur in humanitarian settings compared to settings not affected by crisis. Using interviews conducted by laypeople to distinguish between disorders and severe distress which is not a disorder is difficult in humanitarian settings (for example, interviews carried out by laypeople are unlikely to be able to distinguish between severe, normal grief and a depressive disorder in a recently bereaved person). So, tools used by laypeople (for example, the Self Report Questionnaire, WHO, 1994) can confuse and confound signs of normal distress and mental disorder in humanitarian settings (Bolton & Betancourt, 2004; IASC, 2007; Horwitz, 2007, Rodin & van Ommeren, 2009). This tool aims to side-step this challenge by measuring and reporting symptoms and impaired functioning - without giving a specific diagnosis. Although many decision-makers and community mental health programs would prefer to have data on rates of (probable) mental disorders, data on rates of diverse symptoms of severe distress and functioning are less likely to be disputed and still offer useful descriptive information.

---

[9] Suggested reference: World Health Organization & United Nations High Commissioner for Refugees. WHO-UNHCR Assessment Schedule of Serious Symptoms in Humanitarian Settings (WASSS) (field-test version). In: *Assessing Mental Health and Psychosocial Needs and Resources: Toolkit for Major Humanitarian Settings*. Geneva: WHO, 2012.

Overview

This tool is designed to be used with interviewees 18 years or older living in humanitarian settings. It is also designed to be used at least two weeks after the onset of a crisis.

The tool consists of two independent parts. Part A covers severe, common distress symptoms and impaired functioning in the respondent. Part B includes a broader range of symptoms - including symptoms of psychosis as well as epilepsy - in household members of the respondent. Note that the questions in Part B tend to measure more severe functional impairment than questions in Part A.

Analysis and reporting

As mentioned above, the questions in this tool assess the existence of symptoms of mental distress and functional impairment. Accordingly, you should report on symptoms and not levels of disorders. The easiest way to do this is by reporting percentages of people who responded above a pre-specified threshold on each of the questions. All people that answer 'some of the time', 'most of the time', and 'all of the time' may be grouped into a 'positive (1)' category and other responses as a 'negative (0)' category:

The resulting report would state that:
- X1% of respondents felt **so afraid that nothing could calm them down** most or all of the time in the last 2 weeks.
- X2% of respondents felt **so angry that they felt out of control** most or all of the time in the last 2 weeks.
- X3% of respondents felt **so uninterested in things that they used to like that they did not want to do anything at all** most or all of the time in the last 2 weeks.
- X4% of respondents felt **so hopeless that they did not want to carry on living** most or all of the time in the last 2 weeks.
- X5% of respondents felt **so severely upset about the** emergency/disaster/war **or another event in their life, that they tried to avoid places, people, conversations or activities that reminded them of such event** most or all of the time in the last 2 weeks.
- X6% of respondents felt **unable to carry out essential activities for daily living because of feelings of fear, anger, fatigue, disinterest, hopelessness or upset** most or all of the time in the last 2 weeks.

Source of questions

The phrasing of questions (for example, *'you feel so [emotion] that [consequence]'*) was inspired by the phrasing of some of the WHO World Mental Health Survey's subset of K6 questions (Kessler et al, 2002)[10]. This phrasing is helpful to ensure that the assessment focusses on relatively severe symptoms of distress.

The content of most questions in Part B was inspired by work on indicators of social risk in people with severe mental disorders in Timor Leste (Silove et al, 2004).

---

[10] This phrasing was earlier used in selected items in the Carroll Rating Scale for Depression (Carroll et al, 1981), General Well-Being Scale-RAND (RAND 36-Item Health Survey) (Ware et al, 1979), the Beck Depression Inventory (Beck et al, 1961) and the Taylor Manifest Anxiety Scale (Taylor et al, 1953).

Administration[11]

The average interview time for Part A (six questions) is estimated at two to three minutes. The average time for Part B (assuming an average household of five individuals) is estimated at five minutes.

Before using the tool the interviewer should be trained in general interviewing techniques that are relevant to surveys in humanitarian settings, for example, how to behave ethically and how to probe and avoid introducing bias.

You should use your voice to emphasize all words highlighted in bold in the questions.

'IF NEC' means 'if necessary'. You should prompt the respondent with the response categories, using the truncated wording when specified, until the respondent has learned them well enough to respond without prompting.

'IF VOL' means 'if volunteered'. You should not read these responses out. If the respondent volunteers one of the specified responses, you should record it without additional probing.

Distress during the interview

Thinking about violent or other horrific events can cause people to become distressed. You should not ask details about these events. This is a fully structured tool and specifically designed not to ask for details. If the interviewee wants to talk about these events, you should allow them to do so to some extent, but do not ask them for more details. You should be patient and show that you are listening.

The interviewee may stop the interview at any time. If they ask to stop the interview, you should do this. The person does not need to give a reason for wanting to stop the interview. It is alright to continue with the interview if the person is a little upset and agrees to gently continue with the interview. However, if the person is getting very upset by a topic, you should close the interview booklet and be silent until he or she calms down. You could then say: "You seem very upset. Are you okay to continue the interview or would you prefer to stop?" At the end of the interview, the interviewee should be referred to the best available mental health and psychosocial support worker and you should inform your assessment team leader. Before a first interview you should receive a list of support organisations that you can give to interviewees.

---

[11] Readers are referred to the HESPER manual (WHO & KCL, 2011; http://whqlibdoc.who.int/publications/2011/9789241548236_eng.pdf) for advice on practical and ethical aspects of administering surveys (for example, deciding on the sample size, sampling, recruiting interviewers, setting/privacy, informed consent, managing expectations, ensuring voluntary participation, support for those who may be upset by the interview, reporting frequencies with confidence intervals, and so on.).

References

Beck AT, Ward CH, Mendelson M, Mock J, Erbaugh J. An Inventory for Measuring Depression. *Arch Gen Psychiatry*. 1961;4(6):561-71.

Bolton P, Betancourt TS. Mental health in postwar Afghanistan. *JAMA*. 2004;292:626-8

Carroll BJ, Feinberg M, Smouse PE, Rawson SG, Greden JF. The Carroll rating scale for depression. I. Development, reliability and validation. *Br J Psychiatry*. 1981;138:194-200.

Horwitz AV. Transforming normality into pathology: the DSM and the outcomes of stressful social arrangements. *Journal of Health and Social Behavior* 2007;48: 211-22

Inter-Agency Standing Committee (IASC) *IASC Guidelines on Mental Health and Psychosocial Support in Emergency Settings*. Geneva: IASC, 2007/

Kessler RC, Andrews G, Colpe LJ, Hiripi E, Mroczek DK, Normand SL, Walters EE, Zaslavsky AM. Short screening scales to monitor population prevalences and trends in non-specific psychological distress. *Psychol Med*. 2002 Aug;32(6):959-76.

Rodin D, van Ommeren M. Explaining enormous variations in rates of disorder in trauma-focused psychiatric epidemiology after major emergencies. *International Journal of Epidemiology*. 2009;38:1045-8

Silove D, Manicavasagar V, Baker K, Mausiri M, Soares M, de Carvalho F, Soares A, Fonseca Amiral Z. Indices of social risk among first attenders of an emergency mental health service in post-conflict East Timor: an exploratory investigation. *Aust N Z J Psychiatry*. 2004;38(11-12):929-32.

Taylor JA.. A personality scale of manifest anxiety. *The Journal of Abnormal and Social Psychology*. 1953;48(2): 285-290

Ware JE, Johnston SA, Davies-Avery A. *Conceptualization and Measurement of Health for Adults in the Health Insurance Study: Mental Health*. Rand Corporation: Santa Monica, CA, 1979.

World Health Organization. *A user's guide to the Self-Reporting Questionnaire*. WHO, Geneva, 1994.

World Health Organization & King's College London. *The Humanitarian Emergency Settings Perceived Needs Scale (HESPER): Manual with Scale*. Geneva: World Health Organization, 2011.

PART A	**QUESTIONS TO AND ABOUT THE RESPONDENT. IT IS ASSUMED THAT ESSENTIAL INFORMATION ABOUT THE PERSON (FOR EXAMPLE, SEX, AGE AND SO ON) ARE ESTABLISHED EARLIER IN THE INTERVIEW**

A1. The next questions are about how **you** have been feeling during the **last two weeks**. About how often during the last two weeks did you feel **so afraid that nothing could calm you down** — would you say **all** of the time, **most** of the time, **some** of the time, **a little** of the time, or **none** of the time?

1. ☐	All of the time
2. ☐	Most of the time
3. ☐	Some of the time
4. ☐	A little of the time
5. ☐	None of the time
8. ☐	(IF VOL) Don't know
9. ☐	(IF VOL) Refused

A2. About how often during the last two weeks did you feel **so angry that you felt out of control** — would you say **all** of the time, **most** of the time, **some** of the time, **a little** of the time, or **none** of the time?

1. ☐	All of the time
2. ☐	Most of the time
3. ☐	Some of the time
4. ☐	A little of the time
5. ☐	None of the time
8. ☐	(IF VOL) Don't know
9. ☐	(IF VOL) Refused

A3. During the last two weeks, about how often did you feel **so uninterested in things that you used to like, that you did not want to do anything at all**? (IF NEC: **all** of the time, **most** of the time, **some** of the time, **a little** of the time, or **none** of the time?)

1. ☐	All of the time
2. ☐	Most of the time
3. ☐	Some of the time
4. ☐	A little of the time
5. ☐	None of the time
8. ☐	(IF VOL) Don't know
9. ☐	(IF VOL) Refused

A4. During the last two weeks, about how often did you feel **so hopeless that you did not want to carry on living**? (IF NEC: **all** of the time, **most** of the time, **some** of the time, **a little** of the time, or **none** of the time?)

1. ☐ All of the time 2. ☐ Most of the time	
3. ☐ Some of the time 4. ☐ A little of the time 5. ☐ None of the time	
8. ☐ (IF VOL) Don't know 9. ☐ (IF VOL) Refused	

A5. You may have experienced one or more events that have been intensely upsetting to you, such as the recent emergency/disaster/war.[12] During the last two weeks, about how often did you feel **so severely upset about the emergency/disaster/war or another event in your life, that you tried to avoid places, people, conversations or activities that reminded you of such event**? (IF NEC: **all** of the time, **most** of the time, **some** of the time, **a little** of the time, or **none** of the time?)

1. ☐ All of the time 2. ☐ Most of the time	
3. ☐ Some of the time 4. ☐ A little of the time 5. ☐ None of the time	
8. ☐ (IF VOL) Don't know 9. ☐ (IF VOL) Refused	

A6. The next question is about how these feelings of fear, anger, fatigue, disinterest, hopelessness or upset may have affected you during the last two weeks. During the last two weeks, about how often were you **unable to carry out essential activities** for daily living **because** of these feelings? (IF NEC: **all** of the time, **most** of the time, **some** of the time, **a little** of the time, or **none** of the time?)

1. ☐ All of the time 2. ☐ Most of the time	
3. ☐ Some of the time 4. ☐ A little of the time 5. ☐ None of the time	
8. ☐ (IF VOL) Don't know 9. ☐ (IF VOL) Refused	

---

12 Delete or adapt as relevant to the context.

PART B — (HOUSEHOLD ROSTER QUESTIONS): ONE FORM FOR EACH HOUSEHOLD

	B0A	B0B	B1	B2	B3	B4	B5	B6A	B6B	B7A	B7B
			ASK THESE QUESTIONS ABOUT ALL HOUSEHOLD MEMBERS OLDER THAN 2 YEARS OLD					ASK THESE QUESTIONS ABOUT ALL CHILD HOUSEHOLD MEMBERS BETWEEN 2 AND 12 YEARS OLD		ASK THESE QUESTIONS ABOUT ALL ADOLESCENT/ADULT HOUSEHOLD MEMBERS OLDER THEN 12 YEARS OLD	
						Only ask this question if the response was yes to B3	Only ask this question if the response was yes to B3		Only ask this question if the response was yes to B6A		Only ask this question if the response was yes to B7A
	Age	Sex	During the last 2 weeks, was s/he so distressed/ disturbed/ upset that s/he was **completely inactive or almost completely inactive, because** of any such feelings?	During the last 2 weeks, for how many days was s/he so distressed/ disturbed/ upset that s/he was **unable to carry out essential activities** for daily living, **because** of any such feelings?	Is s/he **acting in strange way or having fits/ convulsions / seizures**?	Could you **describe** in a few words the **fits/ convulsions /seizures or the behaviour** that seems strange to you?	**When** did the strange behaviour start? (Comment: If date unknown, ask whether the behaviour started or increased after the recent emergency)	During the last 2 weeks, did s/he **urinate** at least two times in his/ her bed **during sleep**?	Did s/he have this problem one year ago?	During the last 2 weeks, did s/he **stop caring properly for his/her self** because s/ he is feeling distressed/ disturbed/ upset?	During the last 2 weeks, did s/he **stop caring properly for children** s/he is responsible, because s/ he is feeling distressed/ disturbed / upset?
Who else lives in your household right now? (only ask questions B1-B7 about household members older than 2) 1 = parent 2 = sibling 3 = child 4 = other relative 5 = non-relative	98= don't know 99= refused	1 = male 2 = female	1 = no 2 = yes 8 = don't know 9 = refused	98= don't know 99= refused	1 = no 2 = yes 8= don't know 9 = refused			1 = no 2 = yes 7 = not applicable 8= don't know 9 = refused	1 = no 2 = yes 7 = not applicable 8= don't know 9 = refused	1 = no 2 = yes 7 = not applicable 8= don't know 9 = refused	1 = no 2 = yes 7 = not applicable 8= don't know 9 = refused
☐	☐	☐	☐	☐	☐			☐	☐	☐	☐
☐	☐	☐	☐	☐	☐			☐	☐	☐	☐
etc.											

TOOL 3 — THE HUMANITARIAN EMERGENCY SETTINGS PERCEIVED NEEDS SCALE (HESPER)[13]

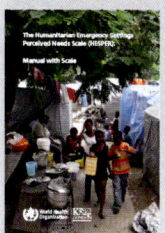

Why use this instrument:: For informing response, through collecting data on the frequency of physical, social, and psychological perceived needs in the community

Method: Community household survey (representative sample) (early in emergencies you can also adapt this method in convenience samples with key informants)

Time needed: 15 to 30 minutes for each interview

Human resources: A HESPER community household survey needs one team leader, between four and eight interviewers and one interviewer supervisor

The HESPER scale provides a quick, scientifically robust way of assessing the **perceived serious needs** of people affected by large-scale humanitarian emergencies (Semrau et al, 2012). Perceived needs are needs which are felt or expressed by people themselves and are problem areas with which they would like help.

The scale assesses a wide range of social, psychological and physical problem areas. It helps quickly identify those broad problem areas with which the population is likely to want help. It needs to be followed by in-depth assessments to understand the expressed needs, and to decide what exact interventions and supports would be helpful. It is possible to disaggregate the results and provide population profiles according to gender, age groups, ethnicity, or other relevant subgroups. The scale focuses on needs as perceived by the adult population.

Perceived needs are assessed on the HESPER scale across 26 needs, which each include a short heading, as well as an accompanying question. Examples of needs include 'Place to live in' ("Do you have a serious problem because you do not have an adequate place to live in?"), 'Education for your children' ("Do you have a serious problem because your children are not in school, or are not getting a good enough education?"), and 'Mental illness in your community' ("Is there a serious problem in your community because people have a mental illness?"). Ratings are then made for each need according to whether:

- it is not being met (that is, it is a serious problem, as perceived by the respondent);
- it is not considered a need (that is, it is not a serious problem, as perceived by the respondent); or
- the respondent didn't answer (that is, declined, not known, or not applicable).

Respondents are also asked to name any unlisted additional needs that are not being met. Among needs that have been rated as unmet, respondents are asked to rank their three most serious problems.

Although the HESPER scale was developed for use in representative samples, you may also use it in convenience samples. This may be appropriate during the first few days or weeks of a large sudden-onset crisis, when representative sampling may not be possible. You can use the scale in acute or chronic humanitarian settings, urban or rural settings, and in camps or communities.

The tool, together with an accompanying operations and training manual, is available at *http://whqlibdoc.who.int/publications/2011/9789241548236_eng.pdf*

---

13 Source WHO & Kings College London. *The Humanitarian Emergency Settings Perceived Needs Scale (HESPER): Manual with Scale.* Geneva, 2011.

TOOL 4	CHECKLIST FOR SITE VISITS AT INSTITUTIONS IN HUMANITARIAN SETTINGS[14]

Why use this tool: For protection and care for people with mental or neurological disabilities in institutions

Method: Site visit, interviews with staff and patients

Time needed: Two hours (for initial impression) and two to three days (for a complete checklist)

Human resources needed: Two people

Background

People with severe mental disorders and other mental and neurological disabilities (including those related to alcohol and other substance use) are at high risk of neglect in humanitarian settings, especially when they live in mental hospitals, social care homes or other institutions. This checklist is useful to collect information to plan humanitarian response to protect and provide basic care for people in institutions.

Your answers to the questions in this tool should be based on a walkabout around the institution and conversations with staff and, where feasible, residents themselves. To minimise bias, it is recommended that the assessment is carried out by two people who should have a different professional background.

When there are only a few hours available for assessing institutions (for example, this situation may arise during the first two weeks of a large sudden-onset emergency) the focus of assessment should be on:

(a) protection issues;
(b) basic survival needs; and
(c) (where relevant) the possibility of evacuation.

The checklist requires you to suggest recommended actions. It is essential that you indicate a time frame for these actions to ensure that the most urgent actions will be implemented first.

Notes

- The term 'resident' is used in the checklist to refer to people living in institutions.
- The QualityRights Tool (WHO, 2012) is the appropriate tool to be used in mental health facilities and social care homes in non-emergency, developmental settings. You should consider using this tool in chronic humanitarian emergencies whenever time and resources are available for an in-depth assessment.

Further reading:

IASC (2007) Guidelines Action Sheet 6.3 on care and protection of people in institutions

---

[14] Suggested reference: World Health Organization & United Nations High Commissioner for Refugees.. Checklist for site visits at institutions in humanitarian settings. In: *Assessing Mental Health and Psychosocial Needs and Resources: Toolkit for Major Humanitarian Settings.* Geneva: WHO, 2012.

GENERAL INFORMATION

Name of institution:		**Activities during visit:**	
Geographical location:			
Interviewer:			
Date and time of visit:			
Length visit:			

Brief description of institution (number of beds, general physical condition):

1. STAFF AND RESIDENTS

1.1	Number of staff who survived the disaster/conflict (crisis)	Psychiatrists:	
		Doctors:	
		Nurses:	
		Psychologists:	
		Social workers:	
		Other staff:	
1.2	Number of staff who died due to the crisis		
1.3	Number of staff who are (still) physically injured due to the crisis		
1.4	Number of staff not attending work during the previous week due to the crisis (for example, because of personal/ family needs)		
1.5	Number of residents who survived the crisis	Total	
		Males:	
		Females:	
		Adults (18 to 65):	
		Elderly (over 65):	
		Adolescents (13 to 17):	
		Children (0 to 12):	
1.6	Number of residents who died due to the crisis		
1.7	Number of residents who are (still) physically injured due to the crisis		
1.8	Number of residents who have left the institution due to the crisis (for example they may have fled or been suddenly discharged)		
1.9	Number of residents with physical disabilities		
1.10	Number of residents with intellectual disabilities		

2. BASIC PHYSICAL NEEDS

2.1 Are water and sanitation facilities adequate? (For example, is there access to clean drinking water, water points and soap)	Action needed: Yes ☐ No ☐ Not applicable/ Don't know ☐
	Resident views/ other comments:
2.2 Is hygiene and personal care adequate (including hygiene facilities and access to personal care items)?	Action needed: Yes ☐ No ☐ Not applicable/ Don't know ☐
	Resident views/ other comments:
2.3 Are food and nutrition adequate? (For example, do residents receive 2 to 3 meals a day that contain adequate nutritional value?)	Action needed: Yes ☐ No ☐ Not applicable/ Don't know ☐
	Resident views/ other comments:
2.4 Are the residents' living and sleeping quarters adequate? (For example, are there enough mattresses, blankets, adequate shelter to protect from weather (heat/cold, rain, wind) and are their quarters clean enough?)	Action needed: Yes ☐ No ☐ Not applicable/ Don't know ☐
	Resident views/ other comments:
2.5 Is physical disease addressed? (Is physical health monitored and is there access to medical care and vaccinations?)	Action needed: Yes ☐ No ☐ Not applicable/ Don't know ☐
	Resident views/ other comments:
2.6 Are physical disability problems addressed? (For example, are facilities accessible and adequate social services available to people with disabilities, and is there help and support from staff when needed such as when using bathroom facilities?)	Action needed: Yes ☐ No ☐ Not applicable/ Don't know ☐
	Resident views/ other comments:

3. MENTAL HEALTH CARE

3.1 Is each resident's mental health status regularly monitored?	Action needed: Yes ☐ No ☐ Not applicable/ Don't know ☐
	Resident views/ other comments:
3.2 Are essential psychotropic medications available?[15]	Action needed: Yes ☐ No ☐ Not applicable/ Don't know ☐
	Resident views/ other comments:
3.3 Are non-pharmacological methods of care (psychosocial rehabilitation, occupational therapy and so on) used?	Action needed: Yes ☐ No ☐ Not applicable/ Don't know ☐
	Resident views/ other comments:

---

15 For a list of essential psychotropic medicines, see Appendix A of IASC Reference Group for Mental Health and Psychosocial Support in Emergency Settings. (2010). Mental Health and Psychosocial Support in Humanitarian Emergencies: What Should Humanitarian Health Actors Know? Geneva. http://www.who.int/mental_health/emergencies/what_humanitarian_health_actors_should_know.pdf

3.4 What is the current staff - resident ratio on the ward?	Action needed: Yes ☐ No ☐ Not applicable/ Don't know ☐
	Resident views/ other comments:
3.5 Do residents have individual treatment files? (For example, files containing case notes which are kept confidentially?)	Action needed: Yes ☐ No ☐ Not applicable/ Don't know ☐
	Resident views/ other comments:

4. PROTECTION ISSUES

4.1 Do children receive care and protection? (For example, safe places to sleep and play, nutrition, stimulation and education?)	Action needed: Yes ☐ No ☐ Not applicable/ Don't know ☐
	Resident views/ other comments:
4.2 Are male and female residents housed separately? (For example, do they have separate quarters for sleeping, and separate latrines/toilets and washing facilities?)	Action needed: Yes ☐ No ☐ Not applicable/ Don't know ☐
	Resident views/ other comments:
4.3 Are there any reports of, or have you witnessed, physical abuse such as beatings as a means of control?	Action needed: Yes ☐ No ☐ Not applicable/ Don't know ☐
	Resident views/ other comments:
4.4 Are there any reports of sexual abuse?	Action needed: Yes ☐ No ☐ Not applicable/ Don't know ☐
	Resident views/ other comments:
4.5 Are there any reports of, or have you witnessed, verbal abuse?	Action needed: Yes ☐ No ☐ Not applicable/ Don't know ☐
	Resident views/ other comments:
4.6 Are any residents physically restrained?	Action needed: Yes ☐ No ☐ Not applicable/ Don't know ☐
	Resident views/ other comments:
4.7 Are any residents locked up?	Action needed: Yes ☐ No ☐ Not applicable/ Don't know ☐
	Resident views/ other comments:
4.8 Are residents neglected?	Action needed: Yes ☐ No ☐ Not applicable/ Don't know ☐
	Resident views/ other comments:

5. EVACUATION	
5.1 Do evacuation plans exist?	Action needed: Yes ☐ No ☐ Not applicable/ Don't know ☐
	Resident views/ other comments:
5.2 Are staff trained in carrying out evacuation plans?	Action needed: Yes ☐ No ☐ Not applicable/ Don't know ☐
	Resident views/ other comments:

6. IMPACT OF CRISIS
Observations on impact of crisis:

7. RECOMMENDED ACTIONS	**BY DATE:**	**BY WHOM:**
7.1		
7.2		
7.3		
7.4		
7.5		
7.6		
7.7		
7.8		
7.9		
7.10		

| TOOL 5 | CHECKLIST FOR INTEGRATING MENTAL HEALTH IN PRIMARY HEALTH CARE (PHC) IN HUMANITARIAN SETTINGS[16] |

Why use this tool: For planning a mental health response in PHC

Method: Site visit, interviews with PHC programme managers and staff

Time needed: One hour for each facility

Human resources needed: One interviewer

Background

Through an interview with clinic managers and staff (key informants), you assess to what extent important psychological and social considerations are and can be addressed in primary health care clinics.

You should integrate assessments of these indicators in general PHC assessments, where possible.

This tool focuses on PHC but it also applies to other general health care settings. The tool focuses on mental disorders but also covers epilepsy, a neurological condition.

For more extensive PHC checklists, please see:
- the International Medical Corps PHC Mental Health Integration Checklist (in preparation); and
- the WHO mhGAP situation analysis checklist (in preparation).

In the tool DK stands for Don't Know; NA stands for Not Applicable

Name/description of facility:	
Size of catchment area:	
Date:	
Interviewer:	
Visit duration:	
Key informant 1: name, position and phone number/email:	
Key informant 2: name, position and phone number/email:	
Key informant 3: name, position and phone number/email:	

---

[16] Suggested reference: World Health Organization & United Nations High Commissioner for Refugees. Checklist for Integrating Mental Health in Primary Health Care in Humanitarian Settings. In: *Assessing Mental Health and Psychosocial Needs and Resources: Toolkit for Major Humanitarian Settings.* Geneva: WHO, 2012.

1. HEALTH INFORMATION SYSTEMS INDICATORS

1.1	Mental disorders are documented in the weekly morbidity report[17]	Yes ☐ No ☐ DK ☐ NA ☐ Comment:

1.2 According to the health information system, in the last two weeks at this clinic, how many people were seen with the following conditions?

1.2.1	depression	____ DK/NA ☐ Comment:
1.2.2	epilepsy	____ DK/NA ☐ Comment:
1.2.3	psychosis	____ DK/NA ☐ Comment:
1.2.4	other mental health problem	____ DK/NA ☐ Comment:

2. WORKER COMPETENCY INDICATORS

2.1 Knowledge of available resources

2.1.1	Health staff know the referral options to the mental health system. (For example, staff know the location, approximate costs and referral procedures for nearby mental health services.)	Yes ☐ No ☐ DK/NA ☐ Comment:
2.1.2	Health staff know available supports (for example, protection agencies/networks, community/social services, community support systems, legal services) offering protection and/or social support for social problems such as domestic violence and rape.	Yes ☐ No ☐ DK/NA ☐ Comment:

2.2 Within the last two years health staff have received training in:

2.2.1	communication skills (for example, active listening, respectful attitude)	Yes ☐ No ☐ DK/NA ☐ Comment:
2.2.2	a basic problem-solving, counselling approach	Yes ☐ No ☐ DK/NA ☐ Comment:
2.2.3	offering basic support to people who are bereaved	Yes ☐ No ☐ DK/NA ☐ Comment:
2.2.4.	offering psychological first aid (that is, basic psychological and social support for people recently exposed to potentially traumatic events)	Yes ☐ No ☐ DK/NA ☐ Comment:

---

17 If mental disorders are documented in the weekly morbidity report, you should ask for copies of this weekly morbidity report for the previous month.

2.3 At least one health care provider at each clinic is competent in identifying and clinically managing:	
2.3.1 depression	Yes ☐ No ☐ DK/NA ☐ Comment:
2.3.2 psychosis	Yes ☐ No ☐ DK/NA ☐ Comment:
2.3.3 epilepsy	Yes ☐ No ☐ DK/NA ☐ Comment:
2.3.4 developmental and behavioural disorders in children and adolescents	Yes ☐ No ☐ DK/NA ☐ Comment:
2.3.5 problems with alcohol use	Yes ☐ No ☐ DK/NA ☐ Comment:
2.3.6 problems with drug use	Yes ☐ No ☐ DK/NA ☐ Comment:
2.3.7 post-traumatic stress disorder	Yes ☐ No ☐ DK/NA ☐ Comment:
2.3.8 acute trauma-induced anxiety that is so severe that it limits basic functioning	Yes ☐ No ☐ DK/NA ☐ Comment:
2.3.9 self-harm/ suicide	Yes ☐ No ☐ DK/NA ☐ Comment:
2.3.10 medically unexplained somatic complaints	Yes ☐ No ☐ DK/NA ☐ Comment:
2.4 Specify what mental health training and clinical supervisions has been received by health staff in the last two years	
General physicians: Nurses: Other staff:	
2.5 What type of clinical supervision arrangements could practically be organised?:	

3. PSYCHOTROPIC MEDICINES

Medicines	Availability in the PHC clinic or nearby pharmacy in the previous two weeks	Specify types available (examples)
3.1 Generic antidepressant medication	☐ Always ☐ Sometimes ☐ Never	(amitriptyline, fluoxetine)
3.2 Generic anti-anxiety medication	☐ Always ☐ Sometimes ☐ Never	(diazepam)
3.3 Generic anti-psychotic medication	☐ Always ☐ Sometimes ☐ Never	(haloperidol, chlorpromazine, fluphenazine)
3.4 Generic anti-epileptic medication	☐ Always ☐ Sometimes ☐ Never	(phenobarbital carbamazepine, diazepam inj, lorazepam inj, phenytoin, valproic acid)
3.5 Generic antiparkinsonian medicine for the management of side effects from antipsychotic medication	☐ Always ☐ Sometimes ☐ Never	(biperiden)

4. REFERRAL INDICATORS

4.1 In the last two weeks PHC clinic received mental-health related referrals *from*:

4.1.1 Mental health specialist care (secondary, tertiary or private care)	Frequently ☐ Sometimes ☐ Never ☐
4.1.2 Community health workers, other community workers, schools, social services and other community social supports, traditional /religious healers	Frequently ☐ Sometimes ☐ Never ☐

4.2 In the last two weeks PHC clinic referred mental-health related referrals *to*:

4.2.1 Mental health specialist care (secondary, tertiary or private care)	Frequently ☐ Sometimes ☐ Never ☐
4.2.2 Community health workers, other community workers, schools, social services and other community social supports, traditional /religious healers	Frequently ☐ Sometimes ☐ Never ☐

5. STAFF AND THEIR WORKLOAD

5.1	Approximate number of general physicians working at any given time in the clinic	_____ DK/NA ☐ Comment:
5.2	Approximate number of general nurses working at any given time in the clinic	_____ DK/NA ☐ Comment:
5.3	Approximate number of other clinical staff (for example, health officers) at any given time in the clinic	_____ DK/NA ☐ Comment:
5.4	Approximate number of patients (with any type of health problem) in the previous week in the clinic	_____ DK/NA ☐ Comment:
5.5	Approximate number of patients (with any type of health problem) seen by general physicians every hour	_____ DK/NA ☐ Comment:

5.6	Approximate number of patients (with any type of health problem) seen by general nurses every hour	_____ DK/NA ☐ Comment:
5.7	Approximate number of community health workers in the catchment area	_____ DK/NA ☐ Comment:

6. WHAT IS THE IMPACT OF THE EMERGENCY/HUMANITARIAN SITUATION ON THE FOLLOWING?

6.1	Number of staff working at any given time at the facility	
6.2	Availability of psychotropic medicines	
6.3	Number of people seeking help for any health problem	
6.4	Number of people seeking help for any mental health problem	

7. SOCIAL INDICATORS

7.1	Health care facility is in safe walking distance of affected community	Yes ☐ No ☐ DK/NA ☐ Comment:
7.2	Furthest distance travelled by patients to access the health facility (in km)	
7.3	The clinic has at least one female health care provider	Yes ☐ No ☐ DK/NA ☐ Comment:
7.4	Each of the local languages is spoken by at least one clinic staff member	Yes ☐ No ☐ DK/NA ☐ Comment:
7.5	Procedures are in place to ensure that patients give consent before major medical procedures	Yes ☐ No ☐ DK/NA ☐ Comment:
7.6	Health care provision is organised in a way that respects privacy (for example, a curtain around consultancy area)	Yes ☐ No ☐ DK/NA ☐ Comment:
7.7	Information about the health status of people and potentially related life events (for example rape, torture) is treated confidentially	Yes ☐ No ☐ DK/NA ☐ Comment:
7.8	PHC care is affordable for all patients	Yes ☐ No ☐ DK/NA ☐ Comment:

8.1 ACCORDING TO THE *KEY INFORMANTS*, WHAT ARE THE THREE MAIN BARRIERS (WITH PROPOSED SOLUTIONS) TO IDENTIFYING AND MANAGING MENTAL DISORDERS IN PHC?

Barrier	Solution
1	
2	
3	

8.2 ACCORDING TO THE *ASSESSOR*, WHAT ARE THE THREE MAIN BARRIERS (WITH PROPOSED SOLUTIONS) TO IDENTIFYING AND MANAGING MENTAL DISORDERS IN PHC?

Barrier	Solution
1	
2	
3	

9. RECOMMENDED ACTIONS ACCORDING TO THE *ASSESSOR*	BY DATE:	BY WHOM:
9.1		
9.2		
9.3		
9.4		
9.5		
9.6		
9.7		
9.8		
9.9		
9.10		

TOOL 6 — NEUROPSYCHIATRIC COMPONENT OF THE HEALTH INFORMATION SYSTEM (HIS)[18]

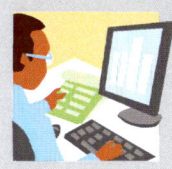

Why use this tool: For advocacy and for planning and monitoring a mental health response in primary health care (PHC)

Method: Clinical epidemiology using the health information system (HIS)

Time needed: Two weeks

Human resources needed: One person

Background

- The PHC HIS must cover mental health. Indeed, one way to rapidly assess frequency of mental health problems and epilepsy is by analysing the HIS.
- The UNHCR HIS includes a 7-category neuropsychiatric component (displayed in Part A below). It is recommended you integrate these seven categories as soon as is possible in the HIS in humanitarian crises.
- Staff will need to be trained (two hours) – and initially supervised (for half a day) in using these categories properly.
- In the UNHCR HIS sex and age data are collected separately and for the following age groups (0 to 4; 5 to17, 18 to 60; over 60)
- Of note, in early days of some acute emergencies, public health decision-makers may not agree on adding 7 items to the HIS. In that situation, at the very least an item labelled "mental, neurological, or substance use problem" may be added to the health information system. Over time this item should then be replaced with the proposed 7 item HIS covered in this Tool.

Category (HIS)	Number seen in last two weeks	Proportion of people seeking help with this problem	2-week treated prevalence
		Divide data in first column by the overall number of patients seen in last two weeks	Divide data in first column by the estimated number of people in catchment area
1. Epilepsy/ seizures			
2. Alcohol or other substance abuse			
3. Mental retardation/ intellectual disability			
4. Psychotic disorder			
5. Severe emotional disorder			
6. Other psychological complaint			
7. Medically unexplained somatic complaint			
Total (sum of 1 to 7)			

---

18 Source for the 7-category HIS described here: United Nations High Commissioner for Refugees (UNHCR). Health Information System (HIS). Geneva: UNHCR, 2009. Reproduced with permission from UNHCR..

CASE DEFINITIONS: NEUROPSYCHIATRIC DISORDERS

1. Epilepsy/seizures
A person with epilepsy has had at least two episodes of seizures not provoked by any apparent cause such as fever, infection, injury or alcohol withdrawal. These episodes are characterised by loss of consciousness with shaking of the limbs and sometimes associated with physical injuries, bowel/bladder incontinence and tongue biting.

2. Alcohol or other substance use disorder
A person with this disorder seeks to consume alcohol (or other addictive substances) on a daily basis and has difficulties controlling how much they consume. Personal relationships, work performance and physical health often deteriorate. The person continues consuming alcohol (or other addictive substances) despite these problems.

3. Mental retardation/ intellectual disability
The person has very low intelligence causing problems in daily living. As a child, this person is slow in learning to speak. As an adult, the person can work if tasks are simple. Rarely will this person be able to live independently or look after themself and/or children without support from others. When severe, the person may have difficulties speaking and understanding others and may require constant assistance.

4. Psychotic disorder
The person may hear or see things that are not there or strongly believe things that are not true. They may talk to themselves, their speech may be confused or incoherent and their appearance unusual. They may neglect themselves. Alternatively they may go through periods of being extremely happy, irritable, energetic, talkative, and reckless. The person's behaviour is considered "crazy"/highly bizarre by other people from the same culture.

5. Severe emotional disorder
This person's daily normal functioning is markedly impaired for more than two weeks due to overwhelming sadness/apathy or exaggerated, uncontrollable anxiety/fear, or both. Personal relationships, appetite, sleep and concentration are often affected. The person may be unable to initiate or maintain conversation. The person may complain of severe fatigue and be socially withdrawn, often staying in bed for much of the day. Suicidal thinking is common.
Inclusion criteria: Only apply this category if there is marked impairment in daily functioning.

CASE DEFINITIONS: OTHER PSYCHOLOGICAL OR MEDICALLY UNEXPLAINED COMPLAINTS OF CLINICAL CONCERN

6. Other psychological complaints
This category covers complaints related to emotions (for example, depressed mood, anxiety), thoughts (for example, ruminating, poor concentration) **or** behaviour (for example, inactivity, aggression). The person tends to be able to function in all or almost all day-to-day, normal activities. The complaint may be a symptom of a less severe emotional disorder or may represent normal distress (that is, no disorder).
Inclusion criteria: Only apply this category if both of the following criteria apply:
- is requesting help for the complaint; **and**
- is not positive for any of the above five categories

7. Medically unexplained somatic complaints
The category covers any somatic/physical complaint that does not have an apparent organic cause.
Inclusion criteria: Only apply this category if all 3 of the following criteria apply:
- after conducting necessary physical examinations;
- if the person is not positive for any of the above six categories; **and**
- if the person is requesting help for the complaint.

TOOL 7 — TEMPLATE TO ASSESS MENTAL HEALTH SYSTEM FORMAL RESOURCES IN HUMANITARIAN SETTINGS[19]

Why use this tool: For planning of (early) recovery/reconstruction, through knowing the formal resources in the regional/national mental health system

Method: Review of documents, interviews with managers of services

Time needed: Three to five days

Human resources needed: One person

Background

Emergencies can be an opportunity for (re)forming nationally available and publicly accessible mental health systems (WHO, in press). An analysis of the formal health system provides essential information for (re)constructing the mental health system after emergencies.

Through consulting secondary information and filling gaps with mental health experts, this tool is intended to identify gaps in formal mental health services.

- Many of these variables (indicators) are adapted from WHO AIMS. For precise definitions of these indicators, see WHO-AIMS 2.2
  http://www.who.int/mental_health/evidence/WHO-AIMS/en/
- Where possible, data should be collected by region and facility
- Where possible and relevant, data about patients should be disaggregated by gender and age (child up to 18, adult 19 to 64, elderly over 65).
- Report data in aggregated format (across the affected area) when findings are not **readily** available in disaggregated format and when time for assessment is limited.

This information is also useful for any post-conflict needs assessment or post-disaster needs assessment that provide facts for large-scale fund-raising events for recovery after very large emergencies.

Sources of information

1. Data from:
   - government
   - MHPSS 4Ws (See Tool 1)
   - WHO-AIMS reports on the country
   - WHO Mental Health Atlas
   - reports by health sector/cluster leads

2. Data from interviews with:
   - government and NGO mental health services programme managers (or health services mangers if no specific mental health service managers exist)
   - health cluster/sector coordinators
   - facilitators of any (cross-cluster/sector) mental health and psychosocial support groups

---

[19] Suggested reference: World Health Organization & United Nations High Commissioner for Refugees. Template to assess mental health system formal resources in humanitarian settings. In: *Assessing Mental Health and Psychosocial Needs and Resources: Toolkit for Major Humanitarian Settings.* Geneva: WHO, 2012.

Impact of the emergency

In the third column, indicate to what extent the emergency has had a negative impact on the functioning of the service.

1. FORMAL MENTAL HEALTH SERVICES IN THE (DEFINED) AREA

1.1 Inpatient psychiatric facilities (both mental hospitals with acute and chronic patients, and acute inpatient wards at general hospital)

Number of facilities		1. No emergency impact (services are fully functioning) ☐ 2. partially functioning *(describe)* ☐ 3. not functioning ☐
Number of beds		
Average number of inpatients a day in the previous month		
Number of psychiatrists		
Number of nurses		
Number of other professional staff (for example, physicians, psychologists, occupational therapists, social workers)		
Estimated % of inpatient units that have psychotropic medicines in each therapeutic category (anti-psychotic, antidepressant, mood stabilizer, anxiolytic, antiepileptic and anti-Parkinsonian) continuously available		

1.2 Outpatient psychiatric facilities (separate between public and private facilities)

Number of facilities		1. No emergency impact (services are fully functioning) ☐ 2. partially functioning *(describe)* ☐ 3. not functioning ☐
Approximate number of people treated in previous month		
Number of psychiatrists		
Number of nurses		
Number of other professional staff (for example, physicians, psychologists, occupational therapists, social workers)		
Number of other staff		
Estimated % of outpatient psychiatry facilities that have psychotropic medicines in each therapeutic category (anti-psychotic, antidepressant, mood stabilizer, anxiolytic, antiepileptic and anti-Parkinsonian) continuously available		

1.3 Other psychological treatment centres (for example NGO services)

Number of centres		1. No emergency impact (services are fully functioning) ☐
Approximate number of people treated in previous month		
Number of psychiatrists		2. partially functioning (describe) ☐
Number of nurses		3. not functioning ☐
Number of psychologists		
Number of social workers		
Number of other professional staff		
Number of other staff		

1.4 Residential facilities and institutions that house people with severe neuropsychiatric disorders

Number of centres		1. No emergency impact (services are fully functioning) ☐
Number of residents with severe mental disabilities		
Number of mental health staff		2. partially functioning (describe) ☐
		3. not functioning ☐

1.5 Other mental health facilities (for example drug and alcohol treatment facilities, homes for children with intellectual disabilities)

Number of centres		1. No emergency impact (services are fully functioning) ☐
Approximate number of people treated in previous month		2. partially functioning (describe) ☐
Number of mental health and substance use staff		3. not functioning ☐

2. MENTAL HEALTH IN GENERAL AND PRIMARY HEALTH CARE CLINICS

2.1 General hospital, general medicine outpatient clinics (without specific focus on psychiatry)

Number of clinics		1. No emergency impact (services are fully functioning) ☐ 2. partially functioning *(describe)* ☐ 3. not functioning ☐
Approximate number of patients (with any type of health problem) seen in the previous week		
Approximate number of patients (with any type of health problem) seen by each physician every hour		
% of clinics that have psychotropic medicines in each therapeutic category continuously available		
Approximate % of clinics with staff providing basic mental health care		

2.2 Primary health care clinics

Number of clinics		1. No emergency impact (services are fully functioning) ☐ 2. partially functioning *(describe)* ☐ 3. not functioning ☐
Approximate number of patients (with any type of health problem) seen in the previous week in each clinic		
Approximate number of patients (with any type of health problem) seen by each physician/nurse every hour		
% of clinics that have psychotropic medicines in each therapeutic category continuously available		
Approximate % of clinics with staff providing basic mental health care		

3. COMMUNITY CARE (CARE BY COMMUNITY HEALTH WORKERS AND COMMUNITY MENTAL HEALTH WORKERS OUTSIDE FACILITIES/ CLINICS)

3.1 Community health workers

Number		1. No emergency impact (services are fully functioning) ☐ 2. partially functioning *(describe)* ☐ 3. not functioning ☐
Average population covered by each worker		
Approximate % of staff involved with basic mental health care		

3.2 Community mental health workers (including community-based rehabilitation workers who work on mental health)

Number		1. No emergency impact (services are fully functioning) ☐ 2. partially functioning *(describe)* ☐ 3. not functioning ☐
Average population covered by each worker		

TOOL 8 — CHECKLIST ON OBTAINING GENERAL (NON-MHPSS SPECIFIC) INFORMATION FROM SECTOR LEADS[20]

Why use this tool: For summarising general (non-MHPSS specific) information already known about the current humanitarian emergency (to avoid collecting more data on what is already known)

Method: Review of available documents

Time needed: One day

Human resources needed: One person

Background

Basic physical needs, education and protection issues are key aspects of the context in which a mental health and psychosocial response occurs. The assessment report should contain at least a paragraph detailing these issues. This information should be available through agencies in the relevant clusters/sectors or on websites, and contacting the relevant lead agencies is likely the quickest way of obtaining key information.

Type of information	Suggested information source	Who to contact	Information received?
1. Population size	Government Overall UN coordinating agency		☐
2. Risk groups	Overall UN coordinating agency		☐
3. Size of risk groups	Overall UN coordinating agency		☐
4. Mortality	Overall UN coordinating agency Health cluster/ sector lead		☐
5. Threats to mortality	Overall UN coordinating agency Health cluster/ sector lead		☐
6. Access to basic needs: food	Nutrition and food security cluster/ sector leads		☐
7. Access to basic needs: shelter	Emergency shelter cluster/ sector lead		☐
8. Access to basic needs: water and sanitation	WAter Sanitation and Hygiene (WASH) cluster/ sector lead		☐
9. Access to basic needs: health care and existing mental health services	Health cluster/ sector lead		☐
10. Access to education	Education cluster/ sector lead		☐
11. Human rights violations and protective frameworks	Protection cluster/ sector lead		☐
12. Social, political, religious, and economic structures and dynamics	Protection cluster/ sector lead		☐
13. Changes in livelihood activities and daily community life	Nutrition cluster/ sector lead Camp coordination/ management cluster/ sector lead Protection cluster/ sector lead Emergency shelter cluster/ sector lead		☐
14. Education and social services, and impact of crisis on these	Education cluster/ sector lead Protection cluster/ sector lead		☐

---

20 Suggested reference: World Health Organization & United Nations High Commissioner for Refugees. Checklist on Obtaining General (non-MHPSS) Information from Sector Leads/Clusters. In: *Assessing Mental Health and Psychosocial Needs and Resources: Toolkit for Major Humanitarian Settings*. Geneva: WHO, 2012.

| TOOL 9 | TEMPLATE FOR DESK REVIEW OF PRE-EXISTING INFORMATION RELEVANT TO MENTAL HEALTH AND PSYCHOSOCIAL SUPPORT IN THE REGION/COUNTRY[21] |

Why use this tool: For summarising mental health and psychosocial support (MHPSS) information about this region/country already known before the current humanitarian emergency (to avoid collecting more data on what is already known)

Method: Literature review

Time needed: Seven to ten days

Human resources needed: Two people

Background

The main part of this tool (part A) consists of a sample table of contents for a desk review.

The table of contents in part A of this tool outlines the major topics for which to summarise existing information, but you need to adapt these to each context. The extent to which you can cover each topic depends on the information available. Different information will be available and important in different humanitarian crises. **Generally you can cover each line of the table of contents in one paragraph in the desk review.**

Often, it will be useful to add to the collected information by interviewing national and international experts. Example questions to ask this group are included in part B which refers to primary data that you could collect to complement data identified though the desk review. If time allows, at least two local experts should read through the review before you finalise it.

You should use the tool flexibly to avoid unnecessary repetition in the resulting report. **It is essential that the report is highly readable by people without advanced academic training so you should avoid jargon and theory**. Where possible, the report should be edited into plain language.

The report should be shared electronically with everyone working on mental health and psychosocial support. And, where relevant, the report should be translated into key local languages.

For a guide on how to conduct literature reviews, see Galvan, J.L. (2006). Writing Literature Reviews: a Guide for Students of the Social and Behavioral and Sciences – 4th Edition. Pyrczak. For an example, see: http://www.who.int/mental_health/emergencies/culture_mental_health_haiti_eng.pdf

---

21 Source: IASC Reference Group on Mental Health and Psychosocial Support in Emergency Settings. Template for Desk Review of Pre-Existing Information Relevant to Mental Health and Psychosocial Support in the Region/Country. In: *IASC Reference Group Mental Health and Psychosocial Support Assessment Guide*, forthcoming. This template has been reproduced here with permission from the IASC Reference Group.

A. SAMPLE TABLE OF CONTENTS OF A LITERATURE REVIEW

1 Introduction
1.1 Rationale for the desk review (description of current/recent emergency)
1.2 Description of methodology used to collect existing information (including any library search terms you used)

2 General context
2.1 Geographical aspects (for example, climate, neighbouring countries)
2.2 Demographic aspects (for example, population size, age distribution, languages, education/ literacy, religious groups, ethnic groups, migration patterns, groups especially at risk to suffer in humanitarian crises)
2.3 Historical aspects (for example, early history, colonisation, recent political history)
2.4 Political aspects (for example, organization of state/ government, distribution of power, contesting sub-groups or parties)
2.5 Religious aspects (for example, religious groups, important religious beliefs and practices, relationships between different groups)
2.6 Economic aspects (for example Human Development Index, main livelihoods and sources of income, unemployment rate, poverty, resources)
2.7 Gender and family aspects (for example, organisation of family life, traditional gender roles)
2.8 Cultural aspects (traditions, taboos, rituals)
2.9 General health aspects
    2.9.1 Mortality, threats to mortality, and common diseases
    2.9.2 Overview of structure of formal, general health system

3 Mental health and psychosocial context
3.1. Mental health and psychosocial problems and resources
    3.1.1 Epidemiological studies of mental disorders and risk/protective factors conducted in the country, suicide rates
    3.1.2 Local expressions (idioms) for distress and folk diagnoses, local concepts of trauma and loss
    3.1.3 Explanatory models for mental and psychosocial problems
    3.1.4 Concepts of the self/ person (for example relations between body, soul, spirit)
    3.1.5 Major sources of distress (for example, poverty, child abuse, infertility)
    3.1.6 Role of the formal and informal educational sector in psychosocial support
    3.1.7 Role of the formal social sector (for example, social services) in psychosocial support
    3.1.8 Role of the informal social sector (for example, community protection systems, neighbourhood systems, other community resources) in psychosocial support
    3.1.9 Role of the non-allopathic health system (including traditional health system) in mental health andpsychosocial support
    3.1.10 Help-seeking patterns (where people go for help and for what problems)
3.2 The mental health system
    3.2.1 Mental health policy and legislative framework and leadership
    3.2.2 Description of the formal mental health services (primary, secondary and tertiary care). Consider the relevant Mental Health Atlas and WHO-AIMS reports among other sources to find out availability of mental health services, mental health human resources, how mental health services are used, how accessible mental health services are (for example distance, fee for service), and the quality of mental health services
    3.2.3 Relative roles of government, private sector, NGOs, and traditional healers in providing mental health care

4 Humanitarian context
4.1 History of humanitarian emergencies in the country
4.2 Experiences with past humanitarian aid in general
4.3 Experiences with past humanitarian aid involving mental health and psychosocial support

5 Conclusion
5.1 Expected challenges and gaps in mental health and psychosocial support
5.2 Expected opportunities in mental health and psychosocial support

6 References

B. DATA TO BE COLLECTED THROUGH INTERVIEWS WITH CULTURAL AND MEDICAL EXPERTS, SOCIAL ANTHROPOLOGISTS, SOCIOLOGISTS, OTHER SOCIO-CULTURAL EXPERTS OR KEY INFORMANTS

Comment: This refers to primary data that you may collect to complement data identified though the desk review

What are the essential concerns, beliefs, and cultural issues that aid providers should be aware of when working on mental health and psychosocial support for [PROVIDE EXAMPLE TARGET GROUP, FOR EXAMPLE PEOPLE WHO SUFFERED LOSSES; FEMALE SURVIVORS OF SEXUAL VIOLENCE]? What actions should be avoided?

[PROBE IF NECESSARY] about the following.
- Local ways of describing emotional difficulties
- Existing resources to cope with emotional difficulties
- Local power structures (for example local hierarchies based on kinship, age, gender, knowledge of the supernatural)
- The political situation (for example issues of favouritism, corruption, instability)
- Interactions between different social groups (for example, ethnic and religious)
- Socially vulnerable or marginalized groups
- Former difficulties or bad experiences with aid agencies
- Gender relations
- Accepting services organised by people from outside the community
- Anything else that aid providers should know

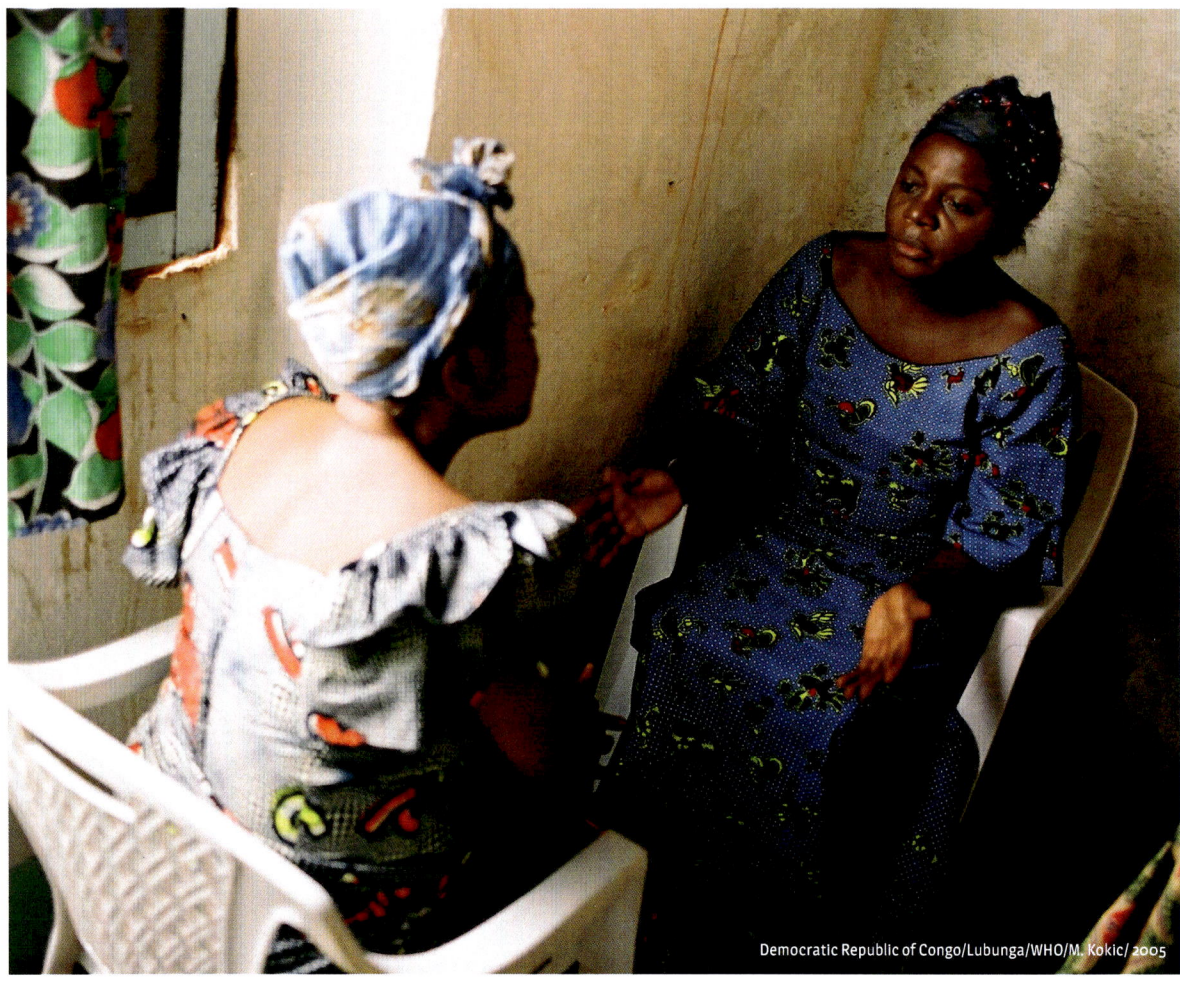

Democratic Republic of Congo/Lubunga/WHO/M. Kokic/ 2005

TOOL 10	PARTICIPATORY ASSESSMENT: PERCEPTIONS BY GENERAL COMMUNITY MEMBERS[22]

Why use this instrument: For learning about local perspectives on problems and coping in a participatory manner, to provide information for MHPSS response

Method: Interviews with general community members (free listing with further questions)

Time needed: One to two days

Human resources needed: Four people

Background

This tool is useful as a way to gain quick information from general community members living in a humanitarian setting.

This tool's first question involves free listing which is often useful in the beginning of an assessment to get an overview of the different types of problems and resources in a community. Free listing means asking an individual (often a general community member) to provide as many answers to a single question as possible. It can focus on a wide variety of topics. For instance, people can be asked to list the types of problems they have, what they do when they face problems, where they go for help and so on.

In the tool described below, the assessor uses free listing to ask respondents about what problems they have. The assessor then selects the type of problem of our interest (that is, mental health and psychosocial problems) for more in-depth assessment on how the problem is seen to impact on daily functioning and how people may cope with it.

You can carry out free listing with individuals or in group settings. However, it is recommended doing it with individuals where feasible, because in a group people may influence each other's answers. It is recommended that you interview at least 10 to 15 people. It may be necessary to interview more than 15 people whenever additional interviews are likely to lead to relevant, new information.

Generally, it will be useful to ask these questions separately for women and men (and for children, youth and adults if this applies) and to check if there are differences.

Before using the tool you should be trained in general interviewing techniques that are relevant to semi-structured interviews in humanitarian settings, for example, how to probe and avoid introducing bias.

---

[22] Source: IASC Reference Group on Mental Health and Psychosocial Support in Emergency Settings. Participatory Assessment I: Perceptions by General Community Members. In: *IASC Reference Group Mental Health and Psychosocial Support Assessment Guide*, forthcoming. This tool has been reproduced here with permission from the IASC Reference Group.

Informed consent

It is important to obtain informed consent before doing any interviews. An example of how to do this is provided here.

> Hello, my name is _____ and I work for _____. We have been working in ___ (area) to _____ (type of work) for ___ (period). Currently, we are talking to people who live in this area. Our aim is to know what kind of problems people in this area have, to decide how we can offer support. We cannot promise to give you support in exchange for this interview. We are here only to ask questions and learn from your experiences. You are free to take part or not.
>
> If you do choose to be interviewed, I can assure you that your information will remain anonymous so no-one will know what you have told us. We cannot give you anything for taking part but we would greatly value your time and responses. Do you have any questions?
>
> Would you like to be interviewed?   1. Yes
>
>   2. No

Interview

Step 1: Free listing

1.1 The interview starts by free listing on the following question to ask for all types of problems.

"What kind of problems do _____ [INSERT GROUP OF INTEREST] have because of the humanitarian situation? Please list as many problems that you can think of."

Notes:

a) Groups of interest may include women in this community, men in this community, teenage girls in this community, young children in this community, etc.

b) When using free listing, you keep on encouraging the respondent to give more answers. For example after the respondent has listed a few problems and remains silent, you could ask:

"What *other* kind of problems do _____ [INSERT GROUP OF INTEREST] have because of the humanitarian situation? Please list as many problems that you can think of." The respondent may now list a few more problems. You would then continue with the question until the respondent gives no more answers.

c) After the list is completed, you should ask for a short description of each problem listed so that the following table can be completed.

TABLE 1. LIST OF PROBLEMS (OF ANY KIND)	
Problem	**Description**
1.1.1	
1.1.2	
1.1.3	
1.1.4	
1.1.5	
1.1.6	
1.1.7	
1.1.8	
1.1.9	
1.1.10	
1.1.11	
1.1.12	
1.1.13	
1.1.14	
1.1.15	
1.1.16	
1.1.17	
1.1.18	
1.1.19	
1.1.20	

1.2 You should then look at the responses to question 1.1 and follow the instructions below to select mental health and psychosocial problems specifically.

Select those problems which are especially relevant from a mental health / psychosocial perspective, such as:

(a) problems related to social relationships (domestic and community violence, child abuse, family separation); and

(b) problems related to:
- feelings (for example feeling sad or fearful);
- thinking (for example worrying); or
- behaviour (for example drinking).

Copy these into Table 1.2 below and also in the first column of Tables 3.1 and 3.2 below.

TABLE 1.2 LIST OF MENTAL HEALTH/PSYCHOSOCIAL PROBLEMS
1.2.1
1.2.2
1.2.3
1.2.4
1.2.5
1.2.6
1.2.7
1.2.8
1.2.9
1.2.10

Step 2: Ranking

2.1 Find out from the respondent which mental health / psychosocial problems are perceived to be important and why.

"You mentioned a number of problems, including [READ OUT PROBLEMS NAMED IN 1.2 ABOVE]. Of these problems, which is the most important problem?" "Why?"

"Of these problems, which is the second most important problem?" "Why?"

"Of these problems, which is the third most important problem?" "Why?"

TABLE 2.1 TOP THREE PRIORITY PROBLEMS		
2.1.1	Problem:	
	Explanation:	
2.1.2	Problem:	
	Explanation:	
2.1.3	Problem:	
	Explanation:	

Step 3: Daily functioning and coping

3.1 Try to identify the impact of mental health / psychosocial problems on daily functioning by asking what tasks could be affected.

"Sometimes [NAME A PROBLEM FROM 1.2 ABOVE] may make it difficult for a person to perform their usual tasks. For example, things they do for themselves, their family or in their community. If a [INSERT GROUP OF INTEREST] suffers from [NAME AGAIN THE PROBLEM LISTED FROM 1.2 ABOVE], what kind of tasks will be difficult for them?"

Report the answer in Table 3.1. Repeat the question for each of the problems mentioned in 1.2.

TABLE 3.1 IMPAIRMENT OF DAILY ACTIVITIES	
Repeat for each problem mentioned under 1.2	
Mental health/ psychosocial problems (as listed in 1.2)	**Affected task**
1.2.1	3.1.1
1.2.2	3.1.2
1.2.3	3.1.3
1.2.4	3.1.4
1.2.5	3.1.5
1.2.6	3.1.6
1.2.7	3.1.7
1.2.8	3.1.8
1.2.9	3.1.9
1.2.10	3.1.10

3.2 Then try to identify how people cope with each of these mental health / psychosocial problems and whether this helps them.

"What kind of things do _____ [INSERT GROUP OF INTEREST] people do to deal with such problems? E.g., things they do by themselves, things they can do with their families or things they do with their communities?" "Does doing that help with the problem?"

Report the answer in Table 3.2. Repeat the question for each of the problems mentioned in 1.2.

TABLE 3.2 COPING		
Repeat for each problem mentioned under 1.2.		
Mental health/ psychosocial problems (as listed in 1.2)	Coping	Is the coping method helpful?
1.2.1	3.2.1	Yes/No
1.2.2	3.2.2	Yes/No
1.2.3	3.2.3	Yes/No
1.2.4	3.2.4	Yes/No
1.2.5	3.2.5	Yes/No
1.2.6	3.2.6	Yes/No
1.2.7	3.2.7	Yes/No
1.2.8	3.2.8	Yes/No
1.2.9	3.2.9	Yes/No
1.2.10	3.2.10	Yes/No

TOOL 11   PARTICIPATORY ASSESSMENT: PERCEPTIONS BY COMMUNITY MEMBERS WITH IN-DEPTH KNOWLEDGE OF THE COMMUNITY[23]

Why use this tool: For learning about local perspectives on problems and coping in a participatory manner, to provide information for MHPSS response

Method: (Individual or group) key informant interviews

Human resources needed: One person

Time needed: Three days for collecting data (assuming the interviewer carries out four interviews a day) and three days for analysis and reporting

Background

This tool is especially useful as a way to gain more in-depth information after preliminary information has been obtained (see Tool 10)

This tool provides questions to use in **key informant or group interviews with community members who are expected to have in-depth knowledge of the affected community**. These could be displacement camp committee members, local staff, religious leaders, traditional healers, women's association leaders, midwives, youth club leaders, school principals, school teachers, counsellors, and so on. You could also include young people.

Do not use all the questions from this tool. Choose those questions that are relevant to you. Remember that a common mistake in assessments is to ask too many questions that are not subsequently analysed, reported or otherwise used. So, do not ask more questions than are needed. Interviews should last no more than one hour. If an interview takes more than one hour, then it is generally better to make a second appointment at another time for a follow-up interview.

When adapting the questionnaire to the local context, **do not** change the sequence of the interview questions (e.g., first asking about problems in a subgroup of the population, then asking what people in this subgroup are doing already to address the problem, and ending with a question on what additional help may be needed)

These interviews can be done with individuals or groups. However, it is recommended to do them with individuals where feasible, because individuals in a group may influence each other's answers. It is recommended to interview at least 10-15 people. It may be necessary to interview more than 15 people whenever additional interviews are likely to lead to relevant, new information.

Before using this tool you should be trained in general interviewing techniques that are relevant to semi-structured interviews in humanitarian settings, for example, how to probe and avoid introducing bias. You should not ask highly sensitive questions that may put people (interviewee, interviewer, or other people) in danger. Depending on the context, these should be asked only during individual key informant interviews (for example questions about people at risk of human rights violations).

---

[23]   IASC Reference Group on Mental Health and Psychosocial Support in Emergency Settings. Participatory Assessment II: Perceptions by community members with in-depth knowledge of the community. In: *IASC Reference Group Mental Health and Psychosocial Support Assessment Guide*, forthcoming. This tool has been reproduced here with permission from the IASC Reference Group.

Remember it can be very relevant to interview traditional/ religious/ indigenous healers on local perceptions of mental health and available resources. A specific tool with questions to interview them is available upon request. That tool in particular is relevant to implementing IASC Guidelines Action 6.4 on potential collaboration with healers.

Informed consent

It is important to obtain informed consent before doing any interviews. An example of how to do this is provided here.

Hello, my name is _____ and I work for _____. We have been working in ___ (area) to _____ (type of work) for ___ (period). Currently, we are talking to people who we believe know a lot about the people affected by this [NAME OF HUMANITARIAN CRISIS, FOR EXAMPLE FLOODS, EXPLOSION, ARMED CONFLICT]. In this interview I would like to ask you about various problems people in the community have. I would also like to ask how people deal with these problems, and if additional help may be needed.

Our aim is to learn from your knowledge and experience, so that we will be better able to provide support. We cannot promise to give you support in exchange for this interview. We are here *only* to ask questions and learn from your experiences. You are free to take part or not.

If you choose to be interviewed, I can assure you that your information will remain confidential. You are free not to take part. We cannot give you anything for taking part but I would greatly value your time and responses. Also, you can stop the interview at any time. Do you have any questions? Would you like to be interviewed?

1. Yes
2. No

A. SOURCES OF DISTRESS

First, I would like to ask you about problems in the community

- What do people in your community believe has caused the current [NAME OF HUMANITARIAN CRISIS, FOR EXAMPLE FLOODS, EXPLOSION, ARMED CONFLICT]?
- According to community members, what are the consequences of the [NAME OF HUMANITARIAN CRISIS, FOR EXAMPLE FLOODS, EXPLOSION, ARMED CONFLICT]?
- According to community members, what will be further consequences of the [NAME OF HUMANITARIAN CRISIS, FOR EXAMPLE FLOODS, EXPLOSION, ARMED CONFLICT]?
- How has the [NAME OF HUMANITARIAN CRISIS, FOR EXAMPLE FLOODS, EXPLOSION, ARMED CONFLICT] affected daily community life?
- How has [NAME OF HUMANITARIAN CRISIS, FOR EXAMPLE FLOODS, EXPLOSION, ARMED CONFLICT] affected people's livelihood, activities/ work?
- How are people trying to rebuild and recover from this crisis?

B. RISK GROUPS

- Which people in your community are suffering the most from the current crisis... Who else?... and who else?

C. NATURE OF DISTRESS AND SUPPORT

C1. Now, I would like to ask a number of questions about children being upset/ distressed.
(COMMENT: You could repeat this question for boys and girls separately and for different age groups, for example, children under 6, children between 6 and 12, and adolescents from 13 to 18).

- How would an outsider recognise a child who is emotionally upset/ distressed by [NAME OF HUMANITARIAN CRISIS, FOR EXAMPLE FLOODS, EXPLOSION, ARMED CONFLICT]?
    a. What does the child look like?
    b. How do they behave?
    c. Are there different types of being upset? What are they?
    d. How can I tell the difference between [NAME ANSWER FROM C1]?
- In normal circumstances (before the recent emergency), what did community members usually do to reduce the upset/ distress of children?
- What are community members doing right now to reduce the upset/ distress of children?
- What else is being done right now to help children who are upset/ distressed?
- Where do children who are upset/ distressed seek help?
- What more could be done to help children who are upset / distressed?

C2. Now, I would like to ask a number of questions about women being upset/ distressed.

- How would an outsider recognize a woman who is emotionally upset/ distressed by the [NAME OF HUMANITARIAN CRISIS, FOR EXAMPLE FLOODS, EXPLOSION, ARMED CONFLICT]?
    a. What does she look like?
    b. How does she behave?
    c. Are there different types of being upset? What are they?
    d. How can I tell the difference between [NAME ANSWER FROM C2]?
- In normal circumstances (before the recent emergency), what did community members usually do for women to reduce upset/ distress?
- What are community members doing for each other right now to reduce women's upset/ distress?
- What else is being done right now to help women who are upset/ distressed?
- Where do women who are upset/ distressed seek help?
- What more could be done to help women who are upset / distressed?

C3. Now, I would like to ask a number of questions about men being upset/ distressed.

- How would an outsider recognize a man who is emotionally upset/ distressed by the [NAME OF HUMANITARIAN CRISIS, FOR EXAMPLE FLOODS, EXPLOSION, ARMED CONFLICT]?
    a. What does he look like?
    b. How does he behave?
    c. Are there different types of being upset? What are they?
    d. How can I tell the difference between [NAME ANSWER FROM C3]?
- In normal circumstances (before the recent emergency), what did community members usually do for men to reduce upset/ distress?
- What are community members doing for each other right now to reduce men's upset/ distress?
- What else is being done right now to help men who are upset/ distressed?
- Where do men who are upset/ distressed seek help?
- What more could be done to help men who are upset / distressed?

C4. Now, I also would like to ask about what happens when people die in your community.

- When someone in this community dies how do the family and friends express their grief?
    a. What are the first things to be done? Why?
    b. How do other family/ friends/ community members express support?
    c. What happens to the body?
    d. What other things need to be done?
    e. How long does mourning continue?
    f. What happens if the body cannot be found/ identified?
- What happens if the process you described (for example, burial) cannot be done?
- What are community members doing for each other right now to helped bereaved families and friends?
- What else is being done right now to help people who are bereaved?
- Where do people who are bereaved seek help?
- What more could be done to help people who are bereaved?

C5. In all communities there are people with mental disorders. May I ask about them? (COMMENT: the word mental disorders may not be well-understood. Where needed, use an appropriate synonym that is understood.)

- Do you have people with mental disorders in the community?
- What kind of problems do they have?
- In general, what do community members think about people with mental disorders? How do they treat them?
- In normal circumstances (before the recent emergency), what did community members usually do to help people with mental disorders?
- What are community members doing right now to help people with mental disorders?
- What else is being done right now to help those with mental disorders?
- Where do people with mental disorders seek help?
- What more could be done to help people with mental disorders?

C6. In most communities there are people (men, women and children) who have been raped or sexually abused. May I ask about them? (COMMENT: additional questions may be phrased by replacing the word 'raped or sexually abused' with 'tortured' or with any other potentially traumatic event that is relevant.)

- If someone has been raped, what kind of problems may the person have?
- In general, what do community members think about people who have been raped? How do they treat them?
- In normal circumstances (before the recent emergency), what did community members normally do to help those who have been raped?
- What are community members doing right now to help those who have been raped?
- What else is being done right now to help those who have been raped?
- Where do people who have been raped seek help?
- What more could be done to help those who have been raped?

C7. In most communities there are people who have problems with alcohol. May I ask about them? (COMMENT: depending on the context, the questions below may need to be asked also - or only - for drugs.)[24]

- If someone frequently drinks a lot of alcohol, what kind of problems may happen in the family or community?
- If someone frequently drinks a lot of alcohol, what kind of problems may happen for him or her?
- In general, what do community members think of people who frequently drink a lot of alcohol? How do they treat them?
- In normal circumstances (before the recent emergency) what did community members normally do to reduce problems caused by alcohol?
- What are community members doing right now to reduce these problems?
- What else is being done right now to deal with these problems?
- Where do people seek help for these problems?
- What more could be done to reduce these problems?

---

24 For a more in-depth tool on alcohol and drug use, see UNHCR & WHO (2008) *Rapid Assessment of Alcohol and Other Substance Use in Conflict-affected and Displaced Populations: A Field Guide*. Geneva: UNHCR."

TOOL 12	PARTICIPATORY ASSESSMENT: PERCEPTIONS BY SEVERELY AFFECTED PEOPLE[25]

Why use this tool: For learning about local perspectives on problems and coping in a participatory manner, to provide information for MHPSS response

Method: Interviews with severely affected people (free listing with further questions)

Time needed: Three to five days

Human resources needed: Two people

This tool provides questions to be used in interviews with people who are severely affected by the humanitarian crisis, for example, because of direct exposure to major trauma or loss.

This tool is useful as a way to gain more in-depth information after preliminary information has been obtained from a desk review (see Tool 9), interviews with general community members (see Tool 10), or interviews with community members with in-depth knowledge of the affected community (see Tool 11). You can use this tool to triangulate data (that is, compare information from different sources).

This first question involves free listing. Free listing means asking an individual to provide as many answers to a single question as possible. It can focus on a wide variety of topics. For instance, you can ask people to list the types of problems they have, what they do when they face problems, where they go for help and so on.

In the example tool described below, you use free listing to ask respondents about what problems they have. You would then select the type of problem of interest (that is, mental health and psychosocial problems) for more in-depth assessment on support and coping.

You can carry out these interviews with individuals or groups. However, it is recommended you do them with individuals where feasible, because individuals in a group may influence each other's answers. It is recommended that you interview at least 10 to 15 people. It may be necessary to interview more than 15 people whenever additional interviews are likely to lead to relevant, new information.

Before using the tool you should be trained in general interviewing techniques that are relevant to semi-structured interviews in humanitarian settings, for example, how to probe and avoid introducing bias.

You should not ask highly sensitive questions that may put people (interviewee, interviewer, or other people) in danger. Depending on the context, these should be asked only during individual key informant interviews (for example questions about people at risk of human rights violations).

Some questions contain probes; you should only use these if necessary (that is, when the respondent cannot think of a response after some time). It is **not** necessary to use each probe one-by-one; they are meant as examples to stimulate a fuller response.

---

25 Suggested reference: World Health Organization & United Nations High Commissioner for Refugees. Participatory Assessment III: Perceptions by severely affected persons themselves. In: *Toolkit for the Assessment of Mental Health and Psychosocial Needs and Resources in Major Humanitarian Settings.* Geneva: WHO, 2012.

Distress

Thinking about violent or other horrific events can cause people to become distressed. You should not probe about these events in detail. This tool is specifically designed not to need a great level of detail. If the interviewee wants to talk about these events, you should allow them to do so to some extent, but you should not ask them for more details as this is not the purpose of doing this assessment. In any case, you should be patient and show that you are listening.

The interviewee may stop the interview at any time. If they ask to stop the interview, you should do this. The person does not need to give a reason for wanting to stop the interview. It is alright to continue with the interview if the person is a little upset but agrees to continue. However, if the person is getting very upset by a topic, you should close the interview booklet and be silent until they calm down. You could then say: "You seem very upset. Are you okay to continue the interview or would you prefer to stop?" At the end of the interview, you should refer the interviewee to the best available psychosocial support worker and you should inform the assessment team leader. Before a first interview you should receive a list of support organisations that you can give to interviewees.

Informed consent

> Hello, my name is _____ and I work for _____. We have been working in ___ (area) to _____ (type of work) for ___ (period). Currently, we are talking with people who live in this area. We would like to talk to you about what kind of problems you are experiencing because of the humanitarian situation, and how you have tried to deal with these.
>
> Our aim is to learn from your knowledge and experience so that we will be better able to provide support. We cannot promise to give you support in exchange for this interview. We are here *only* to ask questions and learn from your experiences. You are free to take part or not. We will use this information to decide how best to support people in similar situations. If you do choose to be interviewed, I can assure you that your information will remain anonymous so no-one will know what you have said. We cannot give you anything for taking part, but we greatly value your time and responses. Do you have any questions? Would you like to be interviewed?
>
> 1. Yes
> 2. No

1. PSYCHOLOGICAL AND SOCIAL DISTRESS

Could you list the problems you are currently experiencing because of the humanitarian situation?

[WHEN THE PERSON STOPS LISTING PROBLEMS, YOU CAN PROBE WITH] What other problems are you currently experiencing because of the humanitarian situation?

[WHEN THE PERSON AGAIN STOPS LISTING PROBLEMS, PROBE WITH] What else? What other problems are you currently experiencing because of the humanitarian situation?

1.1	
1.2	
1.3	
1.4	
1.5	
1.6	
1.7	
1.8	
1.9	
1.10	
1.11	
1.12	
1.13	
1.14	
1.15	

Probe further for psychological and relational problems when the interviewee does not list any mental health or any social issues.

- Have you experienced problems in your relations with other people? If 'yes', what type of problems? [PROBE FURTHER IF NECESSARY. For example, do other people stigmatize you or not give you support? Are you not as involved in community activities as you would like to be?]

- Have you been experiencing problems with your feelings? If 'yes', what type of problems? [PROBE FURTHER IF NECESSARY. For example, do you feel sad or angry or are you afraid?]

- Have you been experiencing problems with the way you think? If 'yes', what type of problems? [PROBE FURTHER IF NECESSARY. For example, do you have problems concentrating, are you thinking too much, are you forgetting things?]

- Have you been experiencing any problems with your behaviour? If 'yes', what type of problems? [PROBE FURTHER IF NECESSARY. For example, are you doing things because you are angry, are you doing things other people have found strange?]

2. SOCIAL SUPPORT AND COPING

I am especially interested in [INSERT ANY RELEVANT PSYCHOSOCIAL AND MENTAL HEALTH PROBLEMS MENTIONED ABOVE].

[FOR EACH PROBLEM OF INTEREST, ASK THE FOLLOWING QUESTIONS]

2.1 Could you tell me how [INSERT PROBLEM] affects your daily life?

2.2 Have you tried to find support for this problem?

2.3 Could you describe how you have tried to deal with this problem? What did you do first? And after that?

2.4 Have you received support from others in dealing with this problem?

2.5 Who gave you this support?

2.6 What kind of support did you get?

2.7 To what extent did this help to deal with the problem?

2.8 Do you feel you need additional support with this problem?

2. SOCIAL SUPPORT AND COPING

Bibliography

Cited publications

Breslau N, Alvarado GF. The clinical significance criterion in DSM-IV post-traumatic stress disorder. *Psychological Medicine* 2007;37:1437-44.

Bolton P, Betancourt TS. Mental health in postwar Afghanistan. *JAMA*, 2004;292: 626-8

Horwitz AV. Transforming normality into pathology: the DSM and the outcomes of stressful social arrangements. *Journal of Health and Social Behavior*. 2007;48: 211-22

Rodin D, van Ommeren M. Explaining enormous variations in rates of disorder in trauma-focused psychiatric epidemiology after major emergencies. *International Journal of Epidemiology*. 2009;38: 1045-8

Semrau M, van Ommeren M, Blagescu M, Griekspoor A, Howard LM, Jordans M, Lempp H, Marini A, Pedersen J, Pilotte I, Slade M, Thornicroft G. The Development and Psychometric Properties of the Humanitarian Emergency Settings Perceived Needs (HESPER) Scale. *Am J Public Health*. 2012; 102(10):e55-e63.

Steel Z, Chey T, Silove D, Marnane C, Bryant R, van Ommeren M. Association of torture and other potentially traumatic events with mental health outcomes among populations exposed to mass conflict and displacement: a systematic review and meta-analysis. *JAMA*, 2009;302:537-49

WHO (2005) *Mental Health Assistance to the Populations Affected by the Tsunami in Asia*. WHO: Geneva.

WHO (in press). *Building back better: Sustainable mental health care after disaster*. Geneva: WHO

Policy documents

Inter-Agency Standing Committee (IASC). *IASC Guidelines on Mental Health nd Psychosocial Support in Emergency Settings*. Geneva: IASC, 2007
http://www.humanitarianinfo.org/iasc/downloadDoc.aspx?docid=4445&ref=4

IASC Global Health Cluster. *Health Cluster Guide: A practical guide for country-level implementation of the Health Cluster*. Geneva: WHO, 2009.
http://www.who.int/hac/global_health_cluster/guide/en/index.html

IASC Reference Group for Mental Health and Psychosocial Support in Emergency Settings. *Mental Health and Psychosocial Support in Humanitarian Emergencies: What Should Humanitarian Health Actors Know?* Geneva, 2010. http://www.who.int/mental_health/emergencies/what_humanitarian_health_actors_should_know.pdf

The Sphere Project. *The Sphere Project: Humanitarian Charter and Minimum Standards in Disaster Response*. Geneva: the Sphere Project, 2011. http://www.sphereproject.org

World Health Organization. *Mental Health in Emergencies: Mental and Social Aspects of Health of Populations Exposed to Extreme Stressors*. Geneva, 2003. http://www.who.int/mental_health/media/en/640.pdf

Ethical guidelines

World Health Organization. *WHO ethical and safety recommendations for researching, documenting and monitoring sexual violence in emergencies.* Geneva, WHO, 2007. http://www.who.int/gender/documents/OMS_Ethics&Safety10Aug07.pdf

Collecting existing mental health systems data

IASC Global Health Cluster: *Health Resources Availability Mapping (HeRAMS).* Geneva: WHO, 2010. http://www.who.int/hac/global_health_cluster/guide/tools/en/index.html

United Nations High Commission for Refugees. *Health Information System (H.I.S).* Geneva, 2009. http://www.unhcr.org/pages/4a30c06f6.html

World Health Organization. *Mental Health Atlas 2011.* Geneva: WHO, 2011. http://www.who.int/globalatlas/default.asp

World Health Organization. *World Health Organization Assessment Instrument for Mental Health Systems 2.2 (WHO-AIMS)* (available in English, French, Russian, Spanish). Geneva: WHO, 2005. http://www.who.int/entity/mental_health/evidence/AIMS_WHO_2_2.pdf

World Health Organization. *WHO-AIMS Country Reports.* Geneva: WHO, 2006-2012. http://www.who.int/mental_health/who_aims_country_reports/en/index.html

Field guides explaining assessment methodology

Active Learning Network for Accountability and Performance in Humanitarian Action. *Participation by Crisis-Affected Populations in Humanitarian Action: a Handbook for Practitioners.* Assessments (Chapter 3) London: Overseas Development Institute, 2003. http://www.alnap.org/pool/files/gs_handbook.pdf

Ager A, Stark L, Potts A, *Participative Ranking Methodology: A Brief Guide (Version 1.1, February 2010).* Program on Forced Migration & Health, Mailman School of Public Health, Columbia University, New York, 2010. http://resources.cpclearningnetwork.org/

Applied Mental Health Research Group. *Design, implementation, monitoring, and evaluation of cross-cultural mental health and psychosocial assistance programs: a user's manual for researchers and program implementers (adult version).* Baltimore: Centre for Refugee and Disaster Response, Johns Hopkins University School of Public Health, in press.

Galvan JL. *Writing Literature Reviews: a Guide for Students of the Social and Behavioral and Sciences – Fourth Edition.* Pyrczak Publishing, 2009.

Health, Nutrition and WASH cluster. *Initial Rapid Assessment (IRA)* (including guidance notes) (draft). Geneva, 2009. http://www.who.int/hac/global_health_cluster/guide/tools/en/index.html

IASC. *The Multi Cluster/Sector Rapid Assessment (MIRA) (provisional version).* IASC: Geneva, 2012. ochanet.unocha.org/p/Documents/mira_final_version2012.pdf

IASC Needs Assessment Task Force. *Operational Guidance for Coordinated Assessments in Humanitarian Crises (Provisional Version February 2011),* 2011. http://oneresponse.info/resources/NeedsAssessment/publicdocuments/Forms/AllItems.aspx

UNHCR, WHO. *Rapid Assessment of Alcohol and Other Substance Use in Conflict-affected and Displaced Populations: A Field Guide.* UNHCR: Geneva, 2008. http://www.who.int/mental_health/emergencies/unhcr_alc_rapid_assessment.pdf

WHO. *QualityRights Toolkit: Assessing and Improve Quality and Human Rights in Mental Health and Social Care Facilities.* WHO, Geneva, 2012

Examples of assessments

Bass J, Poudyal B, Bolton P *An Assessment of the Impact of a Problem-Solving Counseling For Torture-Affected Adults in Aceh, Indonesia, 2008.* Available from: http://pdf.usaid.gov/pdf_docs/PNADU526.pdf

Bolton P. *Qualitative Assessment of Persons affected by torture and related violence in Suleimaniyah Governate, Kurdistan*, Iraq, 2008. Available from: http://pdf.usaid.gov/pdf_docs/PNADP471.pdf

Bolton P, Murray L, Kippen S, Bass J. *Assessment of Urban Street Children and Children living in Government Institutions in Georgia: Development and Testing of a Locally-Adapted Psychosocial Assessment Instrument*, 2007. Available from: http://pdf.usaid.gov/pdf_docs/PNADK676.pdf

HealthNet TPO. *Psychosocial and Mental Health Needs Assessment in Uruzgan, Afghanistan.* Amsterdam: HealthNet TPO, 2009. Available from wietse.tol@yale.edu

International Medical Corps. *IMC Libya Mental Health and Psychosocial Support Assessment Report*, 2011. Available from iweissbecker@InternationalMedicalCorps.org

International Medical Corps. *Displaced Syrians in Za'atari Camp: Rapid Mental Health and Psychosocial Support Assessment: Analysis and Interpretations of Findings*, 2012. Available from iweissbecker@InternationalMedicalCorps.org

Morgan J, Behrendt A. *Silent Suffering: the Psychosocial Impact of War, HIV and other high-risk situations on girls and boys in West and Central Africa.* Working, UK: Plan, 2009. http://www.humansecuritygateway.info/documents/PLANINTL_SilentSuffering_PsychologicalImpactWar_HIV_GirlsBoys_WestCentralAfrica.pdf

Silove D, Manicavasagar V, Baker K, Mausiri M, Soares M, de Carvalho F, Soares A, Fonseca Amiral Z.). Indices of social risk among first attenders of an emergency mental health service in post-conflict East Timor: an exploratory investigation. *Australian and New Zealand Journal of Psychiatry* 2004;38:929-932. http://www.who.int/mental_health/emergencies/silove_indice_of_social_risk.pdf

UNICEF. *The Psychosocial Needs Assessment of Children, Adolescents and Families Affected by the Armed Conflict in Saada Governate.* Yemen: UNICEF, 2007. Available from Almagrami@yahoo.com

WHO. *Five-year mental health plan for northeast Sri Lanka*, 2003. Available from vanommerenm@who.int

WHO/PAHO. *Culture et and Mental Health in Haiti: A Literature Review.* Geneva: WHO, 2010. Available from http://www.who.int/mental_health/emergencies/culture_mental_health_haiti_eng.pdf

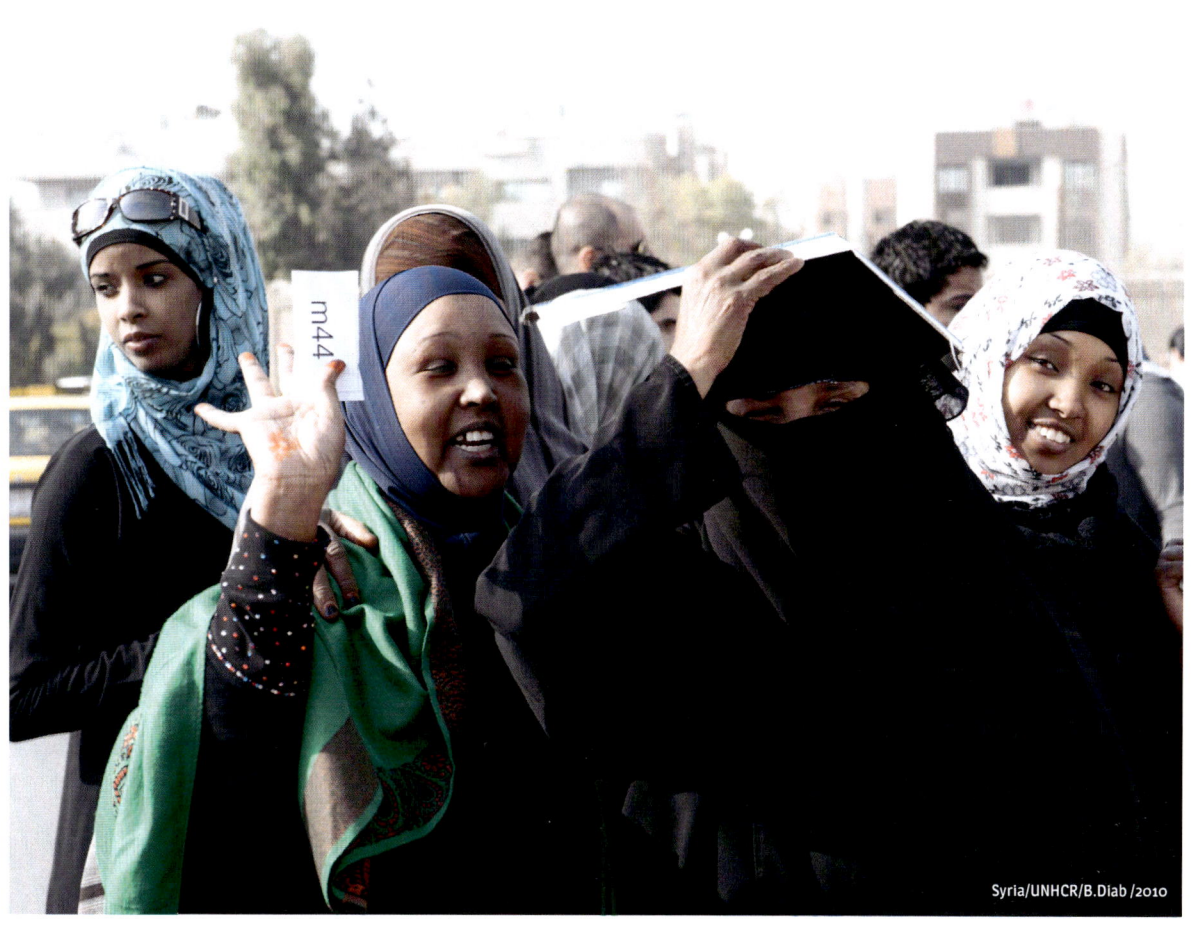

Syria/UNHCR/B.Diab/2010

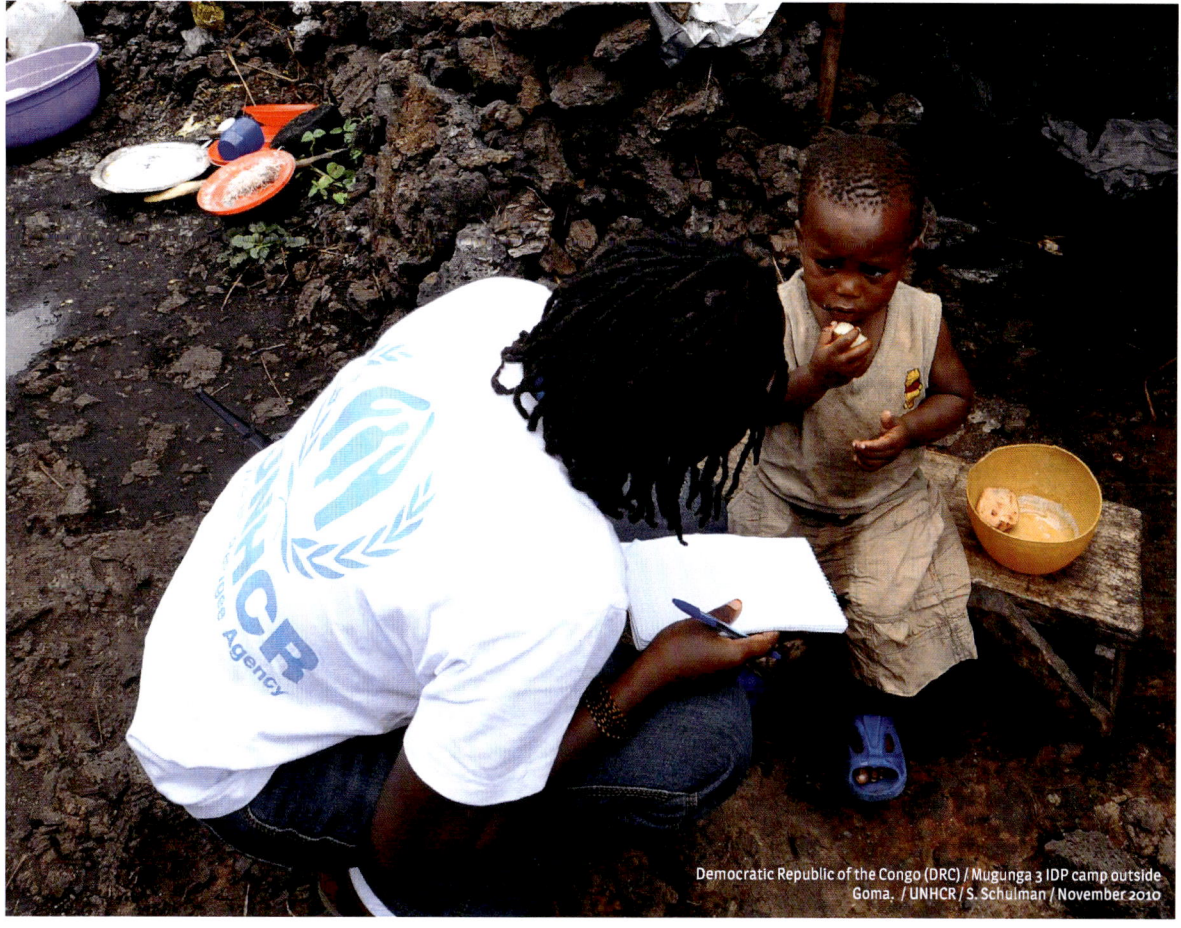

Democratic Republic of the Congo (DRC) / Mugunga 3 IDP camp outside Goma. / UNHCR / S. Schulman / November 2010

A quick guide to identifying tools in this document

Tool #	Title	Method	Why use this tool	Page
For coordination and advocacy				
1	Who is Where, When, doing What (4Ws) in Mental Health and Psychosocial Support (MHPSS): summary of manual with activity codes	Interviews with agency programme managers	For coordination, through mapping what mental health and psychosocial supports are available	30
2	WHO-UNHCR Assessment Schedule of Serious Symptoms in Humanitarian Settings (WASSS)	Part of a community household survey (representative sample)	For advocacy, by showing the prevalence of mental health problems in the community	34
3	Humanitarian Emergency Setting Perceived Needs Scale (HESPER)	Part of a community household survey (representative sample) Or, exceptionally (in acute, major emergencies) as a convenience sample	For informing response, through collecting data on the frequency of physical, social, and psychological perceived needs in the community	41
For MHPSS through health services				
4	Checklist for site visits at institutions in humanitarian settings	Site visits and interviews with staff and patients	For protection and care for people with mental or neurological disabilities in institutions	42
5	Checklist for integrating mental health in primary health care (PHC) in humanitarian settings	Site visits and interviews with primary health care programme managers	For planning a mental health response in PHC	47
6	Neuropsychiatric component of the Health Information System (HIS)	Clinical epidemiology using the HIS	For advocacy and for planning and monitoring a mental health response in PHC	53
7	Template to assess mental health system formal resources in humanitarian settings	Review of documents and interviews with managers of services	For planning of (early) recovery and reconstruction, through knowing the formal resources in the regional/national mental health system	55
For MHPSS through different sectors, including through community support				
8	Checklist on obtaining general (non-MHPSS specific) information from sector leads	Review of available documents	For summarizing general (non-MHPSS specific) information already known about the current humanitarian emergency (to avoid collecting data on issues that are already known)	59
9	Template for desk review of pre-existing information relevant to MHPSS in the region/country	Literature review	For summarizing MHPSS information about this region/country - already known before the current humanitarian emergency (to avoid collecting data on issues that are already known)	60
10	Participatory assessment: perceptions by general community members	Interviews with general community members (free listing with further questions)	For learning about local perspectives on problems and coping to develop an appropriate MHPSS response	63
11	Participatory assessment: perceptions by community members with in-depth knowledge of the community	Interviews with key informants or groups		70
12	Participatory assessment: perceptions by severely affected people	Interviews with severely affected people (free listing with further questions)		74

Note: MHPSS indicates mental health and psychosocial support.